The Raw Facts of Feline Feeding

Alice E. Wright

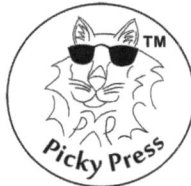

Picky Press

Published by Picky Press

Print ISBN: 9781643949956
EBook ISBN: 9781643949949
Library of Congress Control Number: 2022906196

Our books may be purchased in bulk for promotional, educational, or business use. Contact your local retailer, or contact the author directly at thesiberiancat@yahoo.com.

www.kendersiberiancats.com

Published by Picky Press, an imprint of Tovim Press, LLC. Phoenix, Arizona, USA.

PickyPress.com

Table of Contents

DISCLAIMER

This book was written and published for entertainment and educational purposes. It is in no way meant to replace veterinary care and recommendations. It is always recommended that you consult your trusted holistic or integrative veterinarian for any medical diagnosis or treatment.

The author and publishers disclaim any liability arising from using the materials contained within this book.

Every cat is unique and individual, and requires individual assessment for proper care. This book is not meant to treat, diagnose, or supersede any previously obtained veterinary advice.

Any website, business, organization, cattery, or individual mentioned in this book for reference, is for informational purposes only and does not indicate that the author or publisher or any of their affiliates, support or endorse those named entities. As always, it is the consumer's choice and decision.

Chapter 1
A Raw Intro

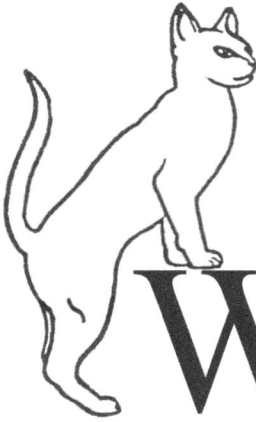

Welcome to *The Raw Facts of Feline Feeding.* Thank you for picking up this book and deciding to give your best to your feline companion through knowledge and growth. I have some axioms for you to read:

1. Cats are obligate carnivores. Not sometimes carnivores, not omnivores, not dogs, not any other kind of animal you want them to be or think them to be. By nature, by design, over the millennia, they are obligate carnivores.

2. Cats, being obligate carnivores, are hunters by their very nature.

Seems simple enough, doesn't it? These are facts that are scientifically not in dispute. Yet many owners, choose to feed a diet not suitable for an obligate carnivore, in effect, treating their beloved pet like something other than the cat she is! But maybe, they weren't aware of what exactly an obligate carnivore is. Or what that term means.

Obligate carnivores are a specialized class of carnivore that solely evolved to eat flesh. They have simpler and shorter digestive tracts than omnivores and herbivores. This streamlined digestive tract is not designed to handle the cell walls of plants. Structure alone tells us the story of a predator with sharp pointed canine teeth for puncturing, grabbing and holding prey, and a mouth full of molars that do not have occlusal tables (horizontal surfaces) used for shearing and tearing. Even a cat's tongue has coarse barbs to help her separate her dinner from its bone. To help facilitate its hunting abilities, all cats come with a set of natural instincts to hunt prey, catch it, and kill it. Whether we throw a ball, play with a feather on a pole, or get her to jump after the red laser dot, we are allowing our kitties to express their natural instincts; albeit in a socially acceptable way. This gives us joy to watch, but also gives your kitty mental enrichment and satisfaction that she just can't get any other way.

They have eyes on the front of their heads pointing forward to help facilitate hunting. They have strong, wide-opening jaws that do not move side to side (which is what herbivores have). They have very sharp pointed teeth that do not line up, to hold, rip and tear their meals, not chew. Cats also lack amylase, an enzyme specifically designed to break down plant cells while chewing. Cats even meet their blood sugar requirements by breaking down the protein in the meat they eat, as opposed to getting it from carbohydrates. Simply put, your cat must eat meat to survive.

As obligate carnivores living in our homes, it is entirely dependent on us to meet the nutritional needs of our kitties.

Dogs are uniquely suited to "make do" as a species, with questionable food sources for short periods of time. As scavenger's and omnivores, this means they can eat many differing types and sources of foods from berries to corn, road kill to even feces. But eventually diet-related health issues show up in the form of allergies, scaly/itchy skin, ear infections, diabetes, kidney and liver disease, and many others. This is also true of cats, except that being obligate carnivores, cats simply cannot "make do" for even short periods of time, which is why we are seeing an escalating number of these diseases in our beloved companions. Cats simply must eat protein sources that they are suited for. Soy, corn, wheat and other "sources" of protein are not in a normal cat's diet.

The feline gastrointestinal tract (GI) is also highly specialized. All animals' GI morphology is primarily influenced by unique adaptations. For cats, this means their stomachs produce a high level of gastric acid to help with breaking down the complex proteins from their diet. Cats have a shorter digestive tract than other species, including dogs and people. For an active predator, this means less weight long-term in the gut to add weight when hunting.

Part of your feeding process must take this faster digestion, shorter GI into consideration. Meals should be no more than 12 hours apart. When more than 12 hours elapses, a cat's stomach can become hyper acidic, causing nausea. And when a cat is nauseated, just like humans, they don't want to eat, which in turn causes more nausea and a cycle begins where veterinary intervention is often required.

All protein is made up from different amino acids and your kitty can only naturally synthesize twelve of these.

The rest of these must come from their diet. The eleven amino acids you must supply for kitty to not only survive but thrive, are arginine, threonine, tryptophan, valine, lysine, isoleucine, leucine, methionine, histidine, phenylalanine, and taurine. The protein in animal tissue has a complete amino acid profile.

Plant-based diets don't contain the correct building blocks for optimal health for our feline friends. Long-term, this can lead to all types of health problems. This is why all commercial pet foods must have nutritional supplementation. This leads to the discussion of dehydration in cats which is much more common than most people believe. Commercial dry pelleted diets do not offer your kitty the moisture they would naturally acquire by eating fresh raw foods.

Domestic cats originated in the arid areas of the Middle East, Egypt, and North Africa. As a result, most cats are less inclined to actively drink from pools or bowls of water. They would naturally get the vast majority of their moisture needs met by eating raw meat. By feeding dry kibble, we are forcing our pets into an unnatural state of chronic dehydration. Cats, unlike dogs, are not efficient at consuming water from outside sources.

Have you ever watched a cat drink? They are lousy drinkers. They often splash and flick it around but their jaws just are not designed to take in large enough quantities of water. By comparison dogs use their tongues like spoons and do a pretty good job of shoveling. Prey species, such as horses and cows can suck large volumes of water very effectively.

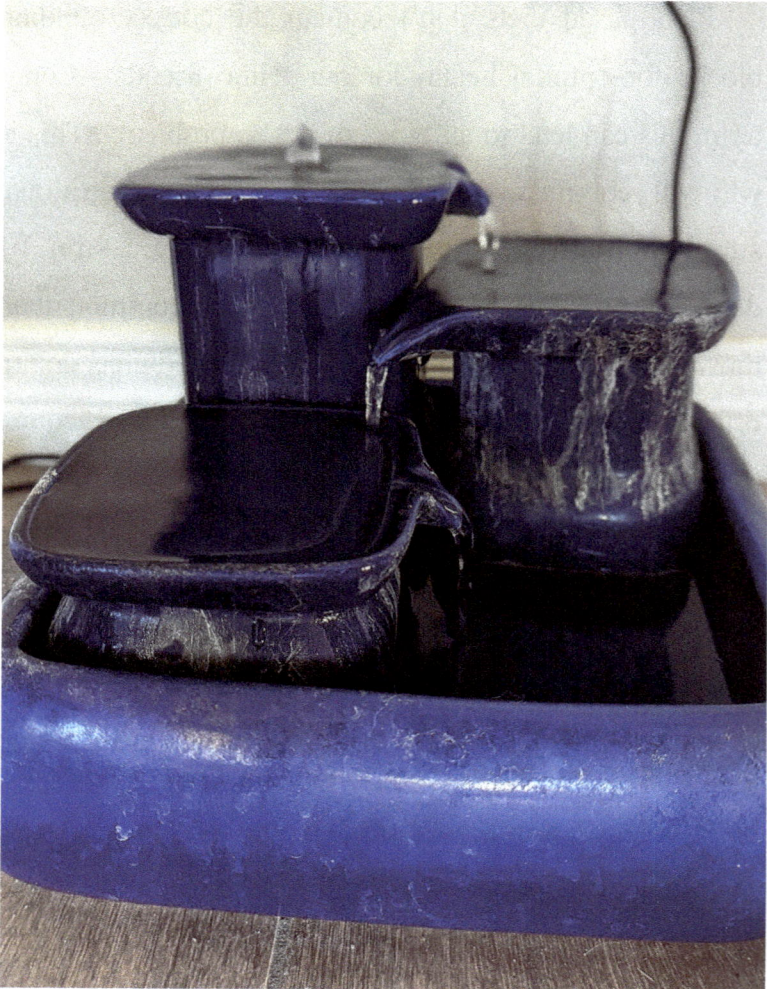

When fed a diet of commercial kibble combined with ineffectual drinking, this often times leads to chronic dehydration. Dehydration puts stress on the kidneys and can lead to cystitis, and even kidney disease in the long term. There are those pesky health issues I brought up earlier. You can help change that by having multiple water vessels available, including bowls, fountains, and even the occasional running tap. Giving foods that are fresh and moist can help minimize this as well.

If you happen to be a breeder feeding a species-appropriate diet, this is critically important to you. Or at least it should be. You see, not only is your cat "what she eats", but so are her offspring and her offspring's offspring. As Kerry J Fowler Msc PhD has said,

"with regard to epigenetics, it (is) worth remembering that the eggs that generate kittens were actually formed in their mother's ovaries when their mother was being formed inside her mother. Therefore, the grandmother's experience in pregnancy can have an epigenetic effect on their daughter's offspring".

What we choose to feed our beloved pets has lasting consequences. There are a staggering number of choices out there today. It is not a topic discussed enough, in my opinion. When you feed a queen (the correct term for a breeding female cat) poorly, you may not see it immediately in her offspring, but you can be sure someone else will see it in her grand kittens. Have a queen who can't give birth naturally or easily? Think about how her mother or grandmother was fed. And this is why choosing to feed your cat like the obligate carnivore she is, is more important than ever.

The goal of feeding your domestic pet is vastly different than the goal of feeding farm animals. We, as concerned, caring pet owners, want to feed the best foods we can afford to ensure our cats have the longest life possible with the greatest health. How do we know that raw feeding is more important than ever? How can our pets tell us that the very food we are giving them is what is making them sick?

Animals can't communicate like us. They don't speak a verbal language. And cats in particular are very good at hiding when they don't feel well. When they throw up continually, have diarrhea, or their tummies hurt, we can't know what they are thinking. Too often, well-meaning veterinarians, behaviorists, pet owners, and even breeders chalk it up to "bad genetics", "poor training", or even old age, because we all know our pets don't live forever. But what if none of that were true? What if the foods we force on our pets are in fact so toxic, so devoid of life-sustaining nutrients, that we are in effect slowly, or even not so slowly, killing our own pets?

The nutritional demands we make of our pet foods is amazing. As humans, we can go out, order in, or make whatever we choose. We have free access to a veritable unlimited supply of differing foods. Then, there are farm animals whose nutrition is solely designed for efficient production, weight gain, and growth, because they rarely live to old age and aren't expected to in our usage and society. There are also our domestic pets– primarily being cats and dogs, whose sole purpose is to live a long and healthy life by our sides. But dogs and cats are essentially "stuck" with whatever comes out of that mass-produced can or bag. They don't have any real choices, even including the time of day they eat. We need to assess this, and ensure that we are meeting the needs of our cats.

When we sit down to eat a meal, we take into account the look of the food. Is it appealing? If we are diabetic, trying to lose weight, or have food allergies or other sensitivities, we have different choices as well.

When we smell the food, we engage our olfactory senses. Our mouths water, and our stomach begins producing acid in anticipation. We might remember a particularly fine meal from the smell, or a family gathering. Maybe even a romantic partner. All of this over one meal. And while our cats aren't human, that doesn't mean they deserve to be fed from a plasticized bag, a single monotonous shape, size and smelling pellet of extruded, rendered garbage.

One of the most important benefits of making your own raw cat food, is that you have choices and control. You pick the primary ingredient in your cat's food. You are guided by your convictions, your lifestyle, and even your budget. The options are limitless, and the value to your pet is immense. You can choose to support organic farmers, raise your own meat, or take advantage of bargains at the supermarket. It is up to you. It's all within your hands.

"An ounce of prevention is worth a pound of cure."

`– Benjamin Franklin

A Discerning Palate

One of the things many folks seem to forget about is taste. We like and dislike certain foods and so do our kitties.

Knowing your pet's anatomy might help you better understand their needs and choices.

Cats have an average number of taste buds, between 450 and 500. This is significantly less than dogs (around 1700), and even less than we humans (around 9000, holy smokes!). Taste receptors are mainly concentrated in two small areas on the tongue called "foliate organs" located at the back of the tongue. The sensation of taste is present as early as five days prior to birth, and improves with age and growth. Cats, like dogs and people can distinguish between the four basic primary taste classifications (sweet, salty, bitter, and sour). However, their sense of taste is diminished due to the smaller number of taste buds. Neurological signals in three cranial nerves are also involved in taste, when stimulated by the taste buds as babies. During the weaning process, when kittens first try their mother's solid food, this is a critical time in terms of influence and experience for developing long-term taste relations and preferences. Kittens are much more likely to attempt a new and novel food when the queen is present, demonstrating how important mom is to a kitten learning good eating habits early. Early weaning, either from loss of the queen or intentional separation, could be a precursor to poor eating habits and food refusal later on. This early learning also may lead to being better able to discern harmful or objectionable foods.

The four basic primary taste classifications are:

- Salty – Generally cats perceive and enjoy food and water enhanced with salt.

- Bitter – Almost always causes an aversion reaction. Cats are more sensitive to bitter than dogs and can detect it at lower levels and is thought to help them avoid common poisons, many of which are bitter.

- Acid – Many commercially available cat food flavors contain phosphoric acid which is widely accepted by more cats. Too much of this along with phosphorus intake, can lead to impaired renal functions.

- Sweet – While cats have the corresponding gene for sweet taste receptors, it appears to have been essentially turned off due to a pseudogene. Generally, cats reject overly-sweet synthetic chemicals such as saccharine and cyclamate and they are perceived by the brain as bitter. It is suspected that the sweet taste of anti-freeze, which appeals to dogs is more a response to their walking through the antifreeze then cleaning their paws and coat. Both are just as deadly of course, but they don't seek it out.

Taste buds for amino acids are connected to the facial nerve and extremely sensitive. It only takes a single amino acid to cause a nerve fiber to react. These adaptations would appear to be a specialization for feeding on amino acid profile-rich raw prey. So, cat food manufacturers have to produce a product that fools the cat's taste palate.

The olfaction (not just the sense of smell but the act or process of smelling) in cats is equally complex. Cats have around 60 to 70 million receptor cells. By comparison, dogs have between 200 and 300 million receptor cells while humans have a mere 50 million receptor cells. Olfaction is *the key* to if a cat will accept a new food or not. If a cat cannot smell a food item, they will not eat that food item. This is why it is critically important that a sick cat, one with a clogged nose, unable to smell, find relief quickly.

Vision is also a key player in your cat's desire to eat. Did you realize that cats cannot see the wavelength between the 520 and 570 nm according to a 1973 study? This means they have a harder time discerning between whites, yellows and greens. But what they may lack in color sense, they more than make up for in their ability to detect movement, as well as having a more panoramic field of vision. These all combine as adaptations to facilitate being an apex predator in their environment.

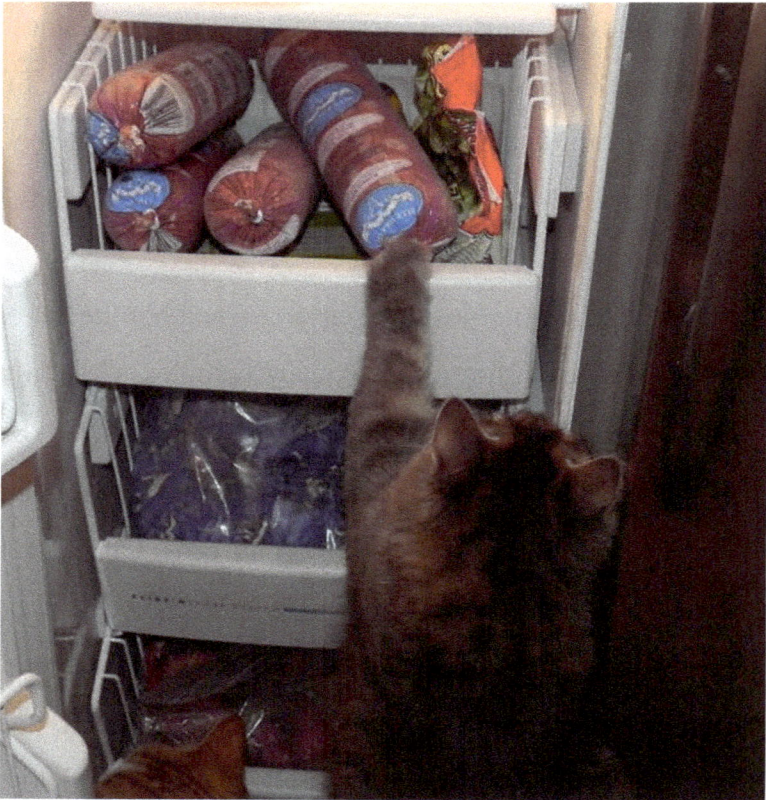

Chapter 2

Introduction to Commercial Cat Foods

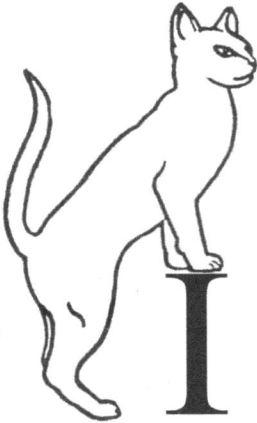

I t may surprise you to know that feeding raw food is not a new or surprising idea. In fact, until very recently, most cats were allowed to roam and hunt their own food in a symbiotic type of relationship with early man. When early man stopped being nomadic and started not only growing but storing grains, cats became a common site and readily ingratiated themselves into our homes and cultures. For cats, this was a great thing.

Here we are, these noisy active bi-pedal things, gathering literal tons of the very food their prey animals desired and sought out. COOL! And the cat subsisted primarily on those attracted rodents and other prey animals. But that was to change sadly, and not for the better.

"If you tell a big enough lie and tell it frequently enough, it will be believed"

– Adolph Hitler

It all began around 1860 in England. An American salesman by the name of James Spratt, had a brainstorm after watching sailors in London throwing leftover "hardtack" to stray and feral dogs on the dock of Liverpool. The creation of Spratt's brainchild became the first ever "Patented Meat Fibrine Dog Cake", or biscuit made exclusively for dogs. And he took this idea and became not only the first to manufacture pet foods, but the first to farm out his production to another company for larger marketing. His "Dog Cakes" were initially sold to English country gentlemen for their sporting dogs and became a status symbol.

CAUTION.—It is most essential that when purchasing you see that every Cake is stamped SPRATT'S PATENT, or unprincipled dealers, for the sake of a trifle more profit, which the makers allow them, may serve you with a spurious and highly dangerous imitation.

GENUINE

SPRATT'S   PATENT

NONE ARE — SPRATTS × PATENT — UNLESS SO

MEAT FIBRINE   DOG CAKES.

STAMPED.

From the reputation these Meat Fibrine Cakes have now gained, they require scarcely any explanation to recommend them to the use of every one who keeps a dog ; suffice it to say they are free from salt, and contain "dates," the exclusive use of which, in combination with meat and meal to compose a biscuit, is secured to us by Letters Patent, and without which no biscuit so composed can possibly be a successful food for dogs.

Price 22s. per cwt., carriage paid; larger quantities, 20s. per cwt., carriage paid.

"Royal Kennels, Sandringham, Dec. 20th, 1873.

" To the Manager of Spratt's Patent.

"Dear Sir,—In reply to your enquiry, I beg to say I have used your biscuits for the last two years, and never had the dogs in better health. I consider them invaluable for feeding dogs, as they insure the food being perfectly cooked, which is of great importance   "Yours faithfully,   C. H. JACKSON."

" 36, North Great George Street, Dublin, June 9th, 1874.

" Gentlemen,—Please to forward to my private residence, as above, 4 cwt. of Dog Biscuits as before ; let them be precisely the same as those supplied on all former occasions   I have much pleasure in bearing personal testimony to their suitability and general efficiency for greyhounds, and in adding that my greyhound, Royal Mary, winner at Altcar of last year's Waterloo Plate, was almost entirely trained for all her last year's engagements upon them.   "Yours obediently,   WILLIAM J. DUNBAR, M.A."

" Rhiwlas, Bala, 21st June, 1873.

" Sir,—I have now tried your Dog Cakes for some six months or so in my kennels, and am happy to be able to give a conscientious testimonial in their favour. I have also found them valuable for feeding horses on a long journey, when strength and stamina are important objects.   It was the opinion of my brother judges and myself that dogs never appeared at the close of a week's confinement in better health and condition than the specimens exhibited at the Crystal Palace Show, and I understand that your Cakes are exclusively used by the manager.   "R. J. LLOYD PRICE."

This concoction of blended wheat meals, vegetables, beetroot and meat, was prepared and baked on the premises of Walker, Harrison and Garthwaite, a firm which then claimed to have baked the first dog biscuit. And an industry was born. Over a very short period of time, Spratt's Dog Cakes were overseas in America and being pushed through billboards, in stores, and even on cigarette cards. It was through this relentless advertising that Spratt's was able to convince the general public who usually fed their dogs table scraps, to buy a product they didn't need.

The company continued to push the snob appeal to hook its customers, even targeting participants and spectators at dog shows, and in 1876 focusing on the centennial exhibition with free food for exhibitors. In January of 1889, the company bought the entire front cover of the first journal of the American Kennel Club in what was obviously a successful attempt to broadcast its involvement with both American and European kennel clubs, and to trumpet the company's "Special Appointment" to Queen Victoria.

In this same publication, they even offer a product for cats in a "pouch" at the amazing price of 1d. And claiming to "entirely supersede the unwholesome practice of feeding on boiled horse flesh..."

In the 1890s, Spratt's products retailed at approximately $7.00–$8.00 per hundredweight and even more for smaller portions. At a time when $1,000-$2,000 was the average annual income for a middle-class American family, this was a princely sum of money.

The company also found new ways to target health-conscious dog owners, and pioneered the concept of animal life stages with so called "appropriate foods" for the various stages. In the 1950s, General Mills acquired Spratt's US business.

As the industry grew, more companies joined in on the
financial boon. Companies like Ken-L-Ration®
introduced canned horse meat for dogs after World War I,

and Gaines Food® introduced canned (or tinned) cat food and dry meat-meal dog food in the 1930s. During World War II, when metal was rationed and pet food was classified as "non-essential", canned pet food wasn't readily available and production shifted to dry kibble foods. After the War, in the 1950s and 60s, when the economy was booming again, people could once again afford the luxury of pet foods. In the 1960s, the industry further diversified with the introduction and production of more varieties of dry (kibble) cat foods and semi-moist products. At this time, canned products for cats, were still mostly fish.

The next big innovation also came in the 1950s with the use of the extrusion process by mass marketers like Purina® (Dog Chow™ and Cat Chow™). The ingredients were liquefied, then cooked together at a high temperature, and then pushed through a mechanical extruder. Think of toothpaste through a tube, all those fun little shapes and colors. This is then baked a second time, again at a high temperature. The extrusion process causes the food, prior to baking, to expand, giving the customer an end-product that is larger and lighter than either of the previous methods. Visually, the food now has a "more for your money" appeal. However, these foods must contain large amounts of starch for the extrusion process to work. And having been cooked two times at high temperatures, additional nutrients have to be added back into the products. Then, often times fats are sprayed onto the outer layer to make the product even palpable to your pet, who can of course smell that. Your pet becomes excited, thus supposedly proving the manufacture's claims of tasty yumminess!

Since 1964 or so, part of the incipient advertising has been the Pet Food Institute's campaign warning consumers about the dangers of feeding table scraps, and the importance of feeding processed food to pets. Marketing soon used terms like "complete" and "guaranteed" with a good housekeeping seal of approval! Clearly, this type of marketing has worked even from the start. Aren't we good little consumers?

In 1968, a company started marketing its pet foods directly to veterinarians and other pet professionals, now known as the famous Hill's Science Diet brand. Their product line continues to expand even today with over 60 of these prescription-only foods marketed exclusively through your veterinary professional. In 1976 the

Colgate-Palmolive Company merged with Riviana Foods, who had previously bought out Hills. Much of the success of their marketing relies on the gullible nature of the public that nutrition is best left to the professionals. Not a bad outcome for a little company that started in 1907 as a rendering plant that had a contract with Topeka, Kansas to dispose of dead and lame animals.

Once the 1970s rolled along, the industry became regulated– or so it is believed. But what really happened was the government allowed the national guidelines for pet nutrition to originate from Ralston Purina's own research department. And what's worse, no one seemed to notice or mind the industry's self-regulation.

In part, this led to the situation where in the 1980s, cat food was found to be lacking what turned out to be essential nutrients, such as taurine. (See Chapter 9 "Let's Get Started".) Pet owners finally *really noticed*, and began actively objecting to their beloved pets getting sick from the very foods being sold as "complete", "balanced" and "nutritious". But what were the results? To understand that, in part, you must also understand the regulatory agencies and their guidelines and mandates.

Chapter 3
The Pottenger Study and Beyond

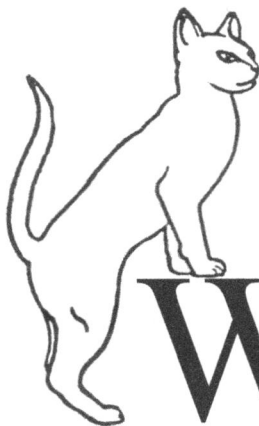

What is truly frustrating is that, between all the mass marketers saying that kibble is the best, veterinarians who are solely educated on nutrition from big brand box companies, and all the so-called experts in the government who really have nothing but printed tables of "facts" to go on, is there really *was* an early study proving beyond a shadow of a doubt that raw is best.

Now all of the naysayers will of course be jumping up and down and screaming in your face, "how dare you contradict them!" But the science is there, and the long-term study is there. The information was published, and it is there. But like all things unpopular, it got buried under an onslaught of propaganda, advertising and people in positions of power who didn't profit from the information.

What may and should astound you, is that this study was no fly-by-night. No looking at other studies and "summarizing" those results. This was an honest-to-goodness, ten-year-long study of over 900 total cats, conducted by a licensed Medical Doctor!

Now admittedly, what this doctor was looking for specifically had to do with his human patients, but the results are what is important for our tiny time in space.

Between 1932 and 1942, Dr. Francis Pottenger conducted a 10-year study in nutrition on 900 cats. What he discovered, was that cats suffered from health complications on a cooked meat diet, and eventually stopped reproducing themselves. Yet in 1948, Morris Sr., founder of Science Diet, ignored Pottenger's findings and proceeded to produce cooked diets. And so, a whole industry began that is still going strong running into the billions of dollars. We, as concerned, caring pet owners, spend every year thinking we are doing our best.

It was reported by the American Pet Products Association (APPA) that in 2020, the US pet-owning population spent $103.6 BILLION. The breakdown looks like this:

🐾 Pet Food & Treats $42.0 billion.

🐾 Supplies, Live Animals & OTC Medicine $22.1 billion.

🐾 Vet Care & Product Sales (think prescription foods) $31.4 billion.

🐾 Other Services $8.1 billion (Other Services include boarding, grooming, insurance, training, pet sitting and walking and all services outside of veterinary care).

According to the AAPA's Pet owners survey, the number of US households that own a cat top a whopping 45 million homes! Every one of those companies spends millions of dollars on advertising to tell you how their product is the do-all and end-all of "special". How Miss Kitty can't live a life of luxury without this new toy, fancy litter, or currently favorable food. And let's face it, "some" companies do get it right. Toys that promote interactive play mimicking Miss Kitty's natural hunting instincts; litter that is both good for her and for your home; and the even rarer raw diet that Miss Kitty needs to not just survive, but thrive.

Clearly the motivation behind the pet industry is profits and not the health of our kitties, which is why it is so important for us as owners to be sure we not only understand what our pets need, but how to make sure they receive it.

Pottenger's study clearly shows us that raw is better and best. We have all heard the mantra to take your vitamins, but that fresh is best. So why is it so hard for us to comprehend that to be true for our kitties as well? Even Harvard Medical School recognizes this. They have been quoted as saying:

> *"The typical American diet is heavy in nutrient-poor processed foods, refined grains, and added sugars—all linked to inflammation and chronic disease."*

(Source: https://www.health.harvard.edu/staying-healthy/ should-you-get-your-nutrients-from-food-or-from -supplements)

Now, why would one of the world's most preeminent educating universities believe this to be true for people? Yet the pet industry continues to push and cram down the public's throat that highly processed refined foods are somehow "safe" to eat, and even going so far as to say:

"In addition, canned pet foods must be processed in conformance with the low acid canned food regulations to ensure the pet food is free of viable microorganisms."

See Title 21 Code of Federal Regulations, Part 113 (21 CFR 113).

There seems to be a complete conflict of interest between maintaining health with fresh foods and an optimal diet, and pushing a highly-processed product that ultimately leads to an unhealthy long-term state.

Pottenger's study readily concluded that cats need to be fed a raw diet to maintain not just their health but the health of their offspring. During the course of the 10-year study, they fed differing types of diets.

The Raw Meat Group

The Raw Meat Group is exactly as it sounds. These cats were fed a diet of 2/3 raw meat, 1/3 raw milk, and added cod liver oil. These cats were, from a scientific standpoint, healthy by displaying clean fur with minimal shedding. They had healthy gums and tissue, and showed no signs of allergies or illness. No susceptibility to fleas or other parasites. From generation to generation, they maintained a regular consistent development and healthy weight, as well as full organ development and normal functions. They had predictable, friendly and outgoing personalities.

The Cooked Meat Group

These cats were fed a diet of 2/3 cooked meats, 1/3 raw milk and added cod liver oil. Heart problems, nearsightedness, under activity of the thyroid gland, infections of the liver and kidneys, arthritis and inflammation were present in all of the cats in this grouping. And by the third generation, they were unable to survive beyond six months of age. Cats in this group showed more irritability and some were even too dangerous to handle.

Within these groups, further study was conducted to include processed foods. Diets were altered to be:

1. 2/3 raw milk, 1/3 raw meat, and cod liver oil.

2. 2/3 pasteurized milk, 1/3 raw meat, and cod liver oil.

3. 2/3 evaporated milk, 1/3 raw meat, and cod liver oil.

4. 2/3 sweetened canned condensed milk, 1/3 raw meat, and cod liver oil.

Cats on the all-raw diet, even though it contained by today's standard something we would never give our cats as a primary source of nutrition, (that being raw milk), fared well. They were generally healthy animals with good coats, nice temperaments, and over all resistant to disease.

The cats fed the pasteurized milk as their principal source of nutrition however, displayed skeletal changes, lessened reproductive efficiency, and their kittens displayed progressive overall health and vitality loss, including chronic respiratory issues.

The third group fed the evaporated milk showed even more severe deficiencies. However, the cats on the sweetened condensed milk were by far the worst off, in terms of health and ability to survive. Even though having large fatty deposits, their overall health was so severely affected as to physically change their skeletal formation. Deformities were common, as was an extreme temperament, irritability displayed by chronic pacing, and nervousness.

In this set of experiments, the cats receiving the pasteurized Vitamin-D milk developed a calcium/ phosphorus imbalance from the normal 2:1 ration to a more than 2.5:1. This caused bone changes to be evidenced and even the development of rickets in some cats. Now why would that be the case if Vitamin-D is the "cure" for rickets in people?

In this case it is a matter of quality vs. quantity. And we go back to, it is a form the body recognizes and can use, called bioavailability. Not all nutrients are created equal, and once heat-processed, most nutrients become so much unusable offal. This is why there is a laundry list of chemical nutrients that must be added back in to all heat-processed foods to make them magically "complete" and "nutritious".

The individual is the product of its past generations; its heredity. And the past generations must be healthy to produce healthy babies. If the grandparents were nutrient-poor, then it can take multiple generations of optimal feeding to see marked improvements in the future generations. And we knew this almost 80 years ago. Raw is best. Fresh is best. Not all forms of food are created equal. So, what happened in between then and now?

> *"Nutrition is the study of health, medicine is the study of disease."*
>
> — Bill Hensley Pharm D.

November 18, 2021. The University of Helsinki has released a focused study showing the distinct correlation between dogs who eat even a partially raw diet having significantly lowered rates of the development of allergy and atopy related skin symptoms in adulthood. The research was published in the Journal of Veterinary Internal Medicine:

> *"The puppies that had been fed raw tripe, raw organ meats, and human meal leftovers during puppyhood showed significantly less allergy and atopy related skin symptoms in adult life. On the other hand, puppies not getting any raw foods, eating most of their food as dry food, i.e. kibble, being fed fruits, and heat-dried animal parts, had*

significantly more allergy and atopy related skin symptoms in adulthood."

"These findings indicate that it was the raw food component that was the beneficial health promotor, and that even as little as 20% of the diet being raw foods, already gives health benefits".

– DogRisk research group team leader, Docent Anna Hielm-Björkman from the Faculty of Veterinary Medicine, University of Helsinki.

We now know and have proof that dogs, who are *not* obligate carnivores, benefit from a raw diet in as little as a 20% of their diet. That dogs, whose jaw structure and gut can eat a wide variety of things, still show marked benefits later in life from a nutritionally complete beginning, which must include raw. Why is that that the pet food industry still feels the need to cook and process and "kill" our pets' food? Why is that obligate carnivores must eat what is clearly not a biologically appropriate diet? And why is it that our so-called experts are still pushing this disease-riddled, disease-causing crap? Would you take a dolphin and feed him a salad? Of course not. So why do people think this is somehow okay for a cat?

Chapter 4

Regulatory Agencies

(That "May" or "May Not" Actually Regulate Your Cat's Food)

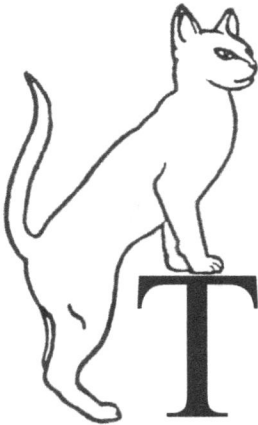

The convoluted "rabbit hole" that is our government's regulatory agencies, will leave even the most die-hard student's head spinning. First, we have the Food and Drug Administration (FDA) which administers and regulates, wait for it... all other agencies that regulate and define your cat's food. Now, within the FDA is an agency called the Center for Veterinary Medicine (CVM). The mission statement for FDA's Center for Veterinary Medicine reads, "Protecting Human and Animal Health". To achieve this broad mission, CVM:

- Makes sure an animal drug is safe and effective before approving it. The center approves animal drugs for companion (pet) animals, such as dogs, cats, and horses; and food-producing animals, such as cattle, pigs, chickens, and even honey bees. If the drug is for a food-producing animal, before approving it, the center also makes sure that food products made from treated animals (meat, milk, eggs, and honey) are safe for people to eat;

- Monitors the safety and effectiveness of animal drugs on the market;

- Makes sure animal food (which includes animal feed, pet food, and pet treats) is safe, made under sanitary conditions, and properly labeled;

- Makes sure a food additive used in animal food is safe and effective before approving it;

- Conducts research that helps the center ensure the safety of animal drugs, animal food, and food products made from animals; and

🐾 Helps make more animal drugs legally available for minor species, such as fish, hamsters, and parrots; and for minor (infrequent and limited) uses in a major species, such as cattle, turkeys, and dogs.

Are we confused yet? You should be. Because this agency claims to monitor animal drugs, yet does not monitor or regulate vaccines. That falls under the purview of the United States Department of Agriculture (USDA). Although it *does* regulate "some" but not all flea and tick products, requiring a six-digit number for production. But don't worry, it doesn't have to be on the label, or at least not until 2023.

Then there is the Federal Food and Cosmetic Act (FFDCA) that regulates... well, foods, drugs, medical devices and cosmetics. And all of this is under the Environmental Protection Act (EPA). Which in turn is what gives the FDA its legal authority to regulate your pet food. Okay, with me so far? Here's where it gets fun.

So, the FFDCA defines the term "food" as "articles used for food or drink for man or other animals", and "articles used for components of any such article." Courts have generally interpreted this to mean a product used primarily for nutrition, taste, or aroma, or components of that product. Then the FFDCA goes on to further define the term "drug" to mean "articles intended for use in the diagnosis, cure, mitigation, treatment, or prevention of disease in man or other animals", and "articles (other than food) intended to affect the structure or function of the body of man or other animals".

Then even beyond that, there is a regulation that states that canned pet food must also comply with the regulations for low-acid canned food.

It's no wonder the common consumer has a hard time finding truth among this nest of vipers. Remember it's all in the marketing. What is generally recognized and considered safe (GRAS) for one usage, may not be GRAS for another. This is particularly true when the fox is monitoring the henhouse! Under FDA's GRAS notification program, companies can make their own GRAS determination, meaning they can determine for themselves if a substance is GRAS for a particular use and then notify the agency of their determination. Of course, there is a procedure and notification process that has to occur for this to be accepted, but who is monitoring all this paperwork and process?

Next, we have the wonderful Dietary Supplement Health and Education Act (DSHEA), which was an amended part of the FFDC Act, in 1994 to create a special category for dietary supplements for people as well as a new regulatory framework for these products. Within this framework, dietary supplements for people fall under the general umbrella of "foods", not drugs or food additives, and as such, the FDA isn't authorized to review dietary supplement products for people for safety or effectiveness before they are marketed. And in 1996 the FDA determined that DSHEA didn't apply to products for use in animals, and at least one court case has upheld the agency's thinking. Therefore, products marketed as dietary supplements for animals don't fall under DSHEA, and the FDA doesn't recognize them. Rather, the agency regulates these products as either food for animals or animal drugs, depending on their intended use.

Now, no one agency can hope to regulate all the human and pet foods, supplements, and drugs that are out there. And here they partner with local, regional and state agencies to enforce a large portion of these mind-numbing regulations. Ready for another acronym?

Part of this "partnering" process is with The Association of American Feed Control Officials (AAFCO). This is a voluntary membership association of local, state and federal agencies. Members are charged by their local, state or federal laws to regulate the sale and distribution of animal feeds, drugs and other remedies.

Did you know?... AAFCO does not regulate, test, approve, or certify pet foods in any way.

AAFCO establishes the nutritional standards for complete and balanced pet foods, and it is the pet food company's responsibility to formulate their products according to the appropriate AAFCO standard.

It is the state feed control official's responsibility in regulating pet food to ensure that the laws and rules established for the protection of companion animals and their custodians are complied with, so that only unadulterated, correctly and uniformly labeled pet food products are distributed in the marketplace and a structure for orderly commerce.

The alphabet soup is thick and heavy, both on paper and in our heads. So, who exactly does regulate what?

Well, here we go again with the alphabet soup wheel of confusion. Within the FDA, the CVM is responsible for the regulation of "animal food (feed) products". It sounds like this entity would set standards for pet foods, but nope! AAFCO, remember them, the volunteer organization almost entirely independent of any governmental control? They actually have this responsibility. The CVM in fact, is only responsible for the regulation of animal drugs, medicated feeds, and food additives. In relation to pet foods, this means that unless a food contains drugs, additives, or makes other health claims, (for example urinary tract health on its label), the CVM, and by extension the FDA, has virtually nothing to do with whether that particular pet food can be sold to the public!

Okay, you say. But what can a "health claim" statement really mean? I mean, a lot of foods out there for felines claim to "lower feline urinary tract disease", "improve coat and skin", or even "reduce shedding and hairballs". These types of statements are considered drug claims, and are generally prohibited by the CVM. Now this sounds like a great idea– yes, let's regulate these sometimes-wild claims by companies, so we don't grow a third eye (okay, extreme idea but you get my point). However, the truth of the matter is a bit different. The CVM by its own wording would seem to discourage these types of claims. But in comes yet another alphabet soup called the Nutrition Labeling and Education Act of 1990 (NLEA), which now requires the FDA to make known the regulations that specifically permit certain health-related claims, on not only human foods, but by extension pet foods as well. So, by incorporating this philosophy into the CVM, they have essentially rolled its proverbial eyes and permitted certain "meaningful" health-related claims on pet food. And this is why we now see such claims as "reduces urine PH to help maintain urinary tract health", and "helps control plaque". Doesn't the word "help" inspire you to confidence? It's supposed to.

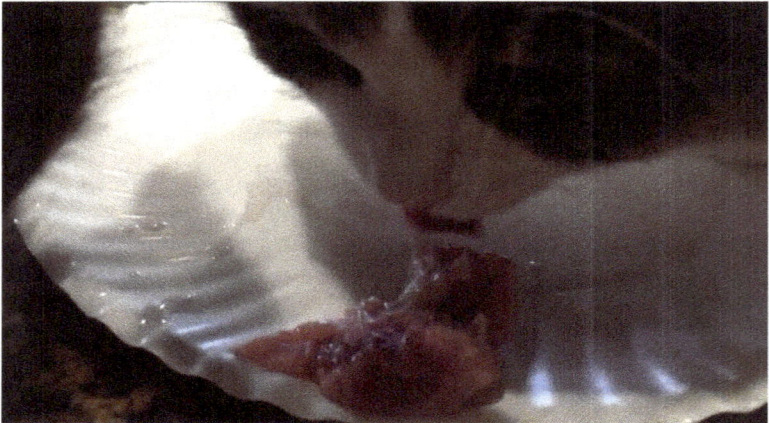

Are you beginning to see why your pet's very health is in the balance?

Congress chose to mandate pet food regulation to the FDA. And the FDA, chooses to focus its attention on human foods and leave the pet foods to other agencies, claiming it is understaffed and overworked. I am sure they are, aren't most governmental agencies?

This void in regulation enforcement then falls on cooperative agreements formed with other groups such as AAFCO. These "feed control officials" first met as an organized committee in 1909. But early feed regulation mainly consisted of protecting the public from a less-than-honest merchant who might be tempted to tip a scale in his favor as opposed to protecting the animals themselves. Now, this agency has grown into a billion-dollar industry right along with pet foods in general. And their reach has grown right along with it. Today, they write feed bills, formulate legislation, control definitions and regulations, along with establish labeling requirements for pet food. AAFCO has no enforcement authority, and performs no testing on the products it oversees. AAFCO's only real requirement is that the manufacturer of the pet food, labels the food according to regulations, staying within the nutritional requirements and ingredient definitions.

For any pet food manufacturer to label a product as nutritionally adequate, they need comply with only one of the following: establish that the product meets the AAFCO's nutrient profiles, perform and meet the feeding trial requirements, or formulate a product that consists of substantially similar components to another food that has already passed an AAFCO feeding trial. Why would a company perform expensive and lengthy feeding trials, when all they have to do is copy someone else? Or, just write up a nutrient profile that passes a standard chemical profile and check all the boxes? Not much of an incentive to produce a quality product.

Did you know that the AAFCO requirement of testing is a grand total of eight, yes, that's right, eight animals?! And that those animals can in fact lose as much as 15% of their individual body weight during this feeding trial. In fact, as long as those eight animals basically don't die during the trial period of only six months (yup, you read that right, *six months*) then the company's food can be sold to you as "complete and balanced"! It doesn't matter if the animals in the trial are unhealthy, lame, itchy, loosing coat etc. What matters is they lived for the whole six months, and that their blood values are within "normal" limits, including hemoglobin, protein and liver enzymes and show no anemia. That's it! Six magical months, and poof they can mass merchandise this product to you. Now that is not to say all companies do this. In fact, many go through lengthy feeding trials and testing well above this bare bones minimum. But it's up to you the consumer to look out and find out which ones are which.

Now we get to the National Research Council's Committee on Animal Nutrition (NRC). Even though the NRC establishes minimum nutrient requirements for growth, based on diets with extremely high digestibility, AAFCO has modified the NRC profiles, under the guise of practicality. Citing AAFCO, specific nutrient requirements were added or modified to support recent scientific publications, practical experience, and unpublished data. Really? Unpublished data? From whom? Seems like a lot of unanswered questions and a mysterious shell game.

But what about that nutrient profile that the AAFCO purports to stand up for and demand? Well, that's all true, 100%. What they *don't* tell you however, is that not all protein and nutrients are created equal to all animals.

This "formulation" method doesn't take into account the bioavailability of any nutrient to the intended target species. Nutrient bioavailability is a much more complex field of study and topic than can successfully be delved into here, beyond just a mere basic understanding.

Bioavailability is the degree that nutrients in your food or your pet's food, are available for absorption and usage by the body. Not everything we eat is utilized by our bodies. These food items become waste materials, processing through our colons and eventually expelled as fecal matter. The same goes for Miss Kitty. We'll discuss this a bit more as we go on. There is a very old story that is rather appropriate to this analogy: "The Animal School," a 1940 fable by George Reavis.

In the fable, a fish goes to a school and is required to work on running and climbing. A duck also is told to improve its running. A rabbit is told to improve its swimming. The goal of the school is to achieve competency results in all subjects, even though this is not physically possible for the various animals. Each animal's unique ability is ignored.

What we see on a daily basis, is that a cat is a dog, is a mouse, is a rat, is a ferret. We feed dog food to cats, and cat food to ferrets and rats. This is grossly inadequate, and is long-term damaging to the individual animals themselves. But how does this all pertain to your cat and the agencies that claim to regulate her foods?

This is where the knowledge of bioavailability becomes useful: What our bodies actually "do" with the items we ingest. In Miss Kitty's case, what she eats. If she is eating bread dough, did you realize some raw yeast could kill her? The yeast can produce alcohol as a byproduct of fermentation. And alcohol is toxic to cats, their livers can't process it. That's also why, although brewer's yeast so popular with dog owners to help prevent fleas and ticks, is also a big "no" for cats. But technically, this is a product also found in many feline products even those specifically marketed to felines. What is truly scary is that even websites like vetinfo.com tout using yeast in your cat's diet. It really shows a lack of understanding your feline's basic structure and design in my opinion. There are many instances in today's so-called cat foods where introduced ingredients are less than stellar and could be downright dangerous long-term.

And what about those pretty bags and cans that prey on our desire to feed the best to our pets by saying "Organic"?

Now, you would think that when a product is labeled as "organic", we as consumers could count on a better quality of pet food. It's definitely a more expensive bag or can of food, but it is no better regulated than anything else. In fact, it is *not regulated at all*. That's right, there are no regulations regarding the labeling of pet foods as organic. None, not one! The AAFCO Official Publication defines the feed term "organic" as a feed or feed ingredient that meets the requirements of the USDA National Organic Program– explained in federal law within Title 7 Code of Federal Regulations Part 205 (7 CFR Part 205). And that sounds great. But with one exception– those regulations are for human food and livestock feed, not pet food. Now, within this 7 CFR Part 205 the word "livestock" is mentioned 95 times, and the word "feed" is included 88 times. However, unlike "feed" laws across almost all US states which define pet food as a feed, the USDA National Organic Program defines feed as: "Edible materials which are consumed by livestock for their nutritional value". But the words "pet" or "pet food" are not mentioned anywhere, not even once. Amazing! And not in a good way.

What is stated on the AAFCO website is that "Organic regulations specific for pet foods are currently being developed." Cool, okay you say, the ball is rolling and it's not being overlooked. Prepare to be disappointed.

In 2004, the National Organic Program organized a task force "to develop labeling standards for organic pet food". Wait...what? 2004? and today it's 2022? Um, what happened? Well, not a whole lot. In 2008 this same task force released their recommendations. Included within their recommendations were labeling requirements of organic pet food such as the requirement for using the words and phrases "organic" or "made with organic" statements on labels. But nothing happened again. Then, in 2010 AAFCO posted on their website an "Update on Organic Pet Foods". Alarmingly, this was not regulatory guidelines but rather the update was from industry itself. The Pet Food Institute to be specific. Within this update it is stated that the National Organic Program shared "that rule-making for pet food will be included in the NOP's priority work plan for FY 2011". But nothing ever happened... again. And to date, no regulations or legal definitions of organic have been accepted of pet food and pet food labeling. So quite literally, all you have is a company's "assurances" that what they say is true. And companies are free to interpret the existing laws based on human foods as they like.

Here is where the alphabet soup of governmental agencies can get even more convoluted. While the National Organic Program is part of the federal USDA, the pet food industry is regulated by sister federal agency FDA. And like most relations, they don't get along. Each tends to regulate within their jurisdiction being careful not cross the line into the other's. Wouldn't want to step on any toes you know. So, while pet foods have AAFCO regulations which are openly accepted by the FDA, the USDA doesn't accept them. Do you have a headache yet?

And here's something else to consider: While the USDA believes that all meat ingredients in pet food should be inspected and passed, the key is the FDA (that actually regulates pet foods) believes condemned meats are suitable for use in pet food. And human grade is in no way organic. But there can be cross-overs in labels. For instance, when pet foods use the words "Human Grade" on the label, these must be manufactured in a licensed human food facility, and have passed the USDA inspections. The organic ingredients in those pet foods would be required to meet the same human food organic regulations. But for a label to just read "organic", don't be fooled. Don't pay a premium for what could be nothing more than labeling.

Chapter 5
Pet Food Since the 1980s

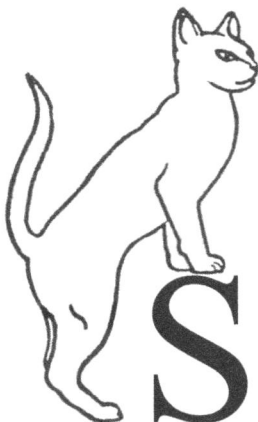

S ince the early 1980s, it would seem that the average pet food consumer is more concerned with quality and becoming educated about ingredients. I mean, it makes sense, right? Beginning in the 1980s were the first mass market home computers, and in 1987 the internet had its birth. So, information from that point forward really shouldn't have been a big secret. Except people really did not educate themselves, and instead let the mass retailers tell them what they should be buying and why. It has become so ingrained in our society that we hardly seem to question it. But clearly, we should have.

Ingredients were not only poor quality, but falsely advertised by many companies. Importing substantially inferior ingredients or purchasing rendered product from questionable sources then-exported for the manufacturing to occur outside the US and other westernized nations led directly to the debacle beginning around 2007/2008.

In March 2007, the FDA learned that certain pet foods were sickening and killing cats and dogs. Surprisingly, the FDA found contaminants in vegetable proteins imported into the United States from China, which were then used as ingredients in pet food manufacturing.

Additionally, some of the tainted ingredients were used to produce farm animal feed and fish feed. The FDA and the US Department of Agriculture also discovered that some animals who ate the tainted feed had then been processed into the human food chain! But don't worry (said tongue-in-cheek) the "government scientists" have determined that there is very low risk to human health from consuming food from animals that ate the tainted feed. Well okay, if they say so it must be true right? Supposedly that tainted pet food, animal and fish feed, and vegetable proteins continue to be recalled and destroyed.

As a result of the FDA and USDA's comprehensive investigation, on February 6, 2008, the FDA announced that two Chinese nationals and the businesses they operated, along with a US company and its president and chief executive officer, were indicted by a federal grand jury for their roles in a scheme to import these products (purported to be wheat gluten) into the United States that were contaminated with melamine. Remember, melamine has been found in the kidneys and urine of cats that died as well as in the food they ate.

What's the big deal with melamine being in your pet's food or even your food? (I mean, besides from being toxic to our cats.) But is it really, or are people just overreacting? Melamine alone may not be the cause of illness and death, because melamine alone is a relatively non-toxic, inert substance. The problem lies when a melamine-related compound cyanuric acid, is also found in pet food. The combination of melamine and cyanuric acid appears to be more toxic than either compound alone. When these two substances interact, they form crystals in the urine and kidney tissues. These two compounds then bind together in the kidney producing extremely fine crystals that arrange themselves in spheres. Those "spherulites" plug the tubules (ureters) transporting urine within the kidney, causing a mechanical obstruction. This obstruction can't be cleared with a food change, because it's all tainted food! The pressure in the kidney builds up, compressing the blood flow to the kidney, causing the cells within the kidney to die and the organ to fail.

Then there is the protein issue. When melamine is added to a product, whether it be milk, baby formula (but that's a whole other discussion), or pet foods, what it does is essentially cut the expense of the product by being a cheap filler. This cheap filler then cuts the actual amount of protein in a product, while at the same time increasing the nitrogen content of the protein. This product therefore appears to have a falsely higher protein content. Think of it this way– a balloon weighs roughly 3 ounces and fits in the palm of your hand. Fill it with water, or air, or any substance, and now it is much too large to fit in your hand, may weigh more, and to the naked eye is literally three, four or more times the size. But did the balloon itself change in its physical make up? It still weighs only 3 ounces. This is only a crude explanation, but I think you get the idea.

Ultimately, melamine was found not only in wheat gluten meal, but rice and rice protein concentrate.

(* And I stress again, neither of these items are digestible to a cat in either case, so they should never have been considered or included in a truly decent food for an obligate carnivore, but here we are).

Over 150 individual brands of cat and dog food (owned and produced by no less than 7 large conglomerate companies) were eventually recalled. Some of the companies include:

- Wilbur-Ellis Feed , who not only manufactures pet food but also ships imported mass quantity pet food ingredients to multiple other companies.

- Natural Balance

- Blue Buffalo

- Menu Foods – another mass production company who produces foods for other companies such as Iams, Eukanuba and store labeled brands

- Colgate-Palmolive

- Hill's – yes the makers of Science Diet

- Del Monte Pet Products

- Nestle Purina Pet Care

"This has exposed that the safety standards for pet foods are not in place in any significant way, and the kind of drumbeat, day after day, of recalls has shaken consumers' confidence in the pet food industry's adherence to food safety standards", said Wayne Pacelle, president and chief executive officer of the Humane Society of the United States.

The House committee even held a food safety hearing to discuss the pet food recall. Finally, the U.S. Attorney for the Western District of Missouri announced that a Nevada company and its owners had entered guilty pleas in federal court "to distributing a tainted ingredient used to make pet food, which resulted in a nationwide recall of pet food and the death and serious illness of countless pets across the United States in 2007." And you would think this would be done and over. But wait, there's more!

In 2006-2007 a multi-state outbreak of the infection Salmonella caused recalls of dry dog and cat foods. Salmonella is something that is zoonotic in nature, meaning we humans can get this. A dog's gut biome is designed to handle various levels of carrion, where as we humans certainly cannot, and can become grievously ill when exposed to the same carrion. Over 70 confirmed cases encompassing 19 states were identified.

Since this time, the FDA has issued recall after recall for pet foods ranging in nature from Listeria, Salmonella, the presence of particulates or foreign matter, and labeling errors, to too much or too little of listed ingredients etc.

Go to the government website: https://www.fda.gov/ animal-veterinary/safety-health/recalls-withdrawals

and you can get an idea of the depth and scope of the problems plaguing the industry.

In addition to recalls, there are even lawsuits between companies alleging false advertising claims based on product analysis. In 2018, a case was adjudicated against the California company, "Wilbur-Ellis Feed LLC" (remember them from the melamine recalls) for admitting to substituting lower-cost ingredients for premium, (more expensive chicken and turkey meal in shipments from a plant in Rosser, Texas), to pet food manufacturers between June 2013 and May 2014. On one or more occasions, the plea says, that the lower cost product was hydrolyzed poultry feathers or hydrolyzed feather meal, which consists of ground-up feathers. The pet feed ingredient broker "Diversified Ingredients" involved in the incident (middle-man between ingredient supplier and pet food manufacturer) also pled guilty. So now, we have an importer and broker both acknowledging to have sold feathers rendered into a powder, as a premium meat product. (From a news article by writer Robert Patrick, and dated May 23, 2018.)

McAtee, a trader, broker and co-owner of Diversified Ingredients Inc. of Ballwin, admitted in his plea that the pet food companies that were his company's clients received adulterated and misbranded pet food ingredients from the Rosser facility between 2012 and May 2014. One client received the ingredients between 2012 and May 2014, his plea says. Other companies, which were not identified in the plea but which made and packed food for Blue Buffalo, received multiple adulterated shipments between 2012 and May of 2014. McAtee removed the word "blend" from some documents, and forged signatures of a Wilbur-Ellis employee on forms to conceal the source or contents of shipments, his plea says.

Chapter 6
A Pet-Eats-Pet World

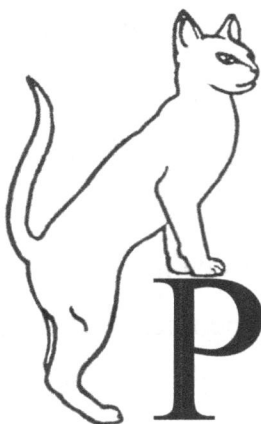

Pets Eating Pets. The Following Information is NOT for the Faint of Heart. You Have Been Warned!

"Nutrition is the study of health, Medicine is the study of disease."
– Bill Hensley Pharm D.

Yup, you read that right. Did you know that for decades, a good number of low-end processors have been picking up and rendering our deceased pet dogs and cats? Is it possible that we have all been feeding our beloved cats and dogs the rendered remains of other cat and dogs?

Isn't that a gruesome thought? Shades of "Soylent Green".

Remember what the FDA does? They are charged with protecting the public's health. They do this, ostensibly through ensuring the safety of the foods we eat as well as our pets. Now, no one can or should claim that they have perfected the system. Especially in light of what happens to the ingredients that don't qualify for human consumption. The ingredients that have been proven to cause cancer, or are known to be bad for the body. These ingredients then find their way into these huge rendering plants that service multiple pet food manufacturers. These ingredients that we know cause incurable cancers in people, diabetes, nutrient deficiencies, thyroid disease, kidney disease and even death, are suddenly magically transformed, or "rendered" into acceptable ingredients for pet foods.

From a 1995 EPA document, it is extensively detailed about these processes that these ingredients go through, including collection and consolidation.

Plants that collect their raw materials from a variety of offsite sources are called "independent rendering plants". Independent plants obtain animal by-product materials, including grease, blood, feathers, offal, and entire animal carcasses, from the following sources: butcher shops, supermarkets, restaurants, fast-food chains, poultry processors, slaughterhouses, farms, ranches, feedlots, and animal shelters.

This document clearly lists animal shelters as sources of material for these rendering plants. Now think about this. How did those animals die? Surely it wasn't old age. Of course, sadly some are hit by cars or other unknown injuries, heat exposure, freezing or dehydration. But what about the others? Was there cancer or open wounds involved? Weren't they euthanized with a chemical cocktail? Pentobarbital is the single most commonly used drug to euthanize our domestic animals.

In 2002, the FDA put out a FOIA (Freedom of Information Act) notice that in part reads:

> *"During the 1990s, FDA's Center for Veterinary Medicine (CVM) received reports from veterinarians that pentobarbital, an anesthetizing agent used for dogs and other*

animals, seemed to be losing its effectiveness in dogs. Based on these reports, CVM officials decided to investigate a plausible theory that the dogs were exposed to pentobarbital through dog food, and that this exposure was making them less responsive to pentobarbital when it was used as a drug."

Well, if it's in dog food, you know it's in cat food! This notice goes on to say:

"Because in addition to producing anesthesia, pentobarbital is routinely used to euthanize animals, the most likely way it could get into dog food would be in rendered animal products.

Rendered products come from a process that converts animal tissues to feed ingredients. Pentobarbital seems to be able to survive the rendering process. If animals are euthanized with pentobarbital and subsequently rendered, pentobarbital could be present in the rendered feed ingredients."

This very statement would lead you to conclude that your pet dogs and cats are clearly and knowingly being processed into the very foods that are being fed back to your dogs and cats!

The CVM scientists then created a test that was to detect DNA of cats and dogs from all the samples of the latest survey materials dated 2000. This method is believed to detect a minimum of 5 pounds of rendered remains in 50 tons of finished feed. And consequently, it was assumed that the pentobarbital residues are entering pet foods that came from euthanized, rendered cattle or even horses. CVM even went on and designed a study using measured doses of phenobarbital in dogs for eight weeks. After the eight weeks, they determined that there was no observable-effect for pentobarbital found in the pet food. Sounds good, doesn't it? The government found a problem, conducted a study, and determined it wasn't a problem. But here's "the problem" or rather the multitude of problems:

🐾 The study was only conducted over eight weeks. In other words, just a mere two months. I don't know about you, but I sure hope my pet lives longer than two months!

🐾 There is never a number of dogs named in the study. Obviously, there is a control group dog and then the three study group dogs, so at least we know there were four dogs tested. I don't know about you, but four dogs out of the US population of over 89 million pet dogs seems rather slim pickings, and not the least bit representative. Maybe there were more, but who knows.

🐾 Pentobarbital is only licensed for use in dogs, not sheep, not cattle, not horses, and is strictly regulated by not only the FDA, but the DEA as well! Even the pet food industry's article of 2018 acknowledges this fact, as well as it being cost-prohibitive to use on such large animals.

🐾 Sharon Gilbert (author of *The Armageddon Strain*, and whose education includes theology, molecular biology, and genetics) has been quoted as saying "DNA is a very delicate molecule (chain). It is true that DNA is destroyed when it is exposed to extreme heat. If the rendering plant in question had in fact, applied high degrees of heat during the rendering process, then it is highly likely that the DNA from any dog or cat would be destroyed and therefore be undetectable in subsequent DNA testing of the animal feed."

🐾 Zero tests or testing on or for cats! Go back to axiom number 1, cats are not dogs! What kills a cat doesn't bother a dog and what kills a dog might not bother a cat. So, 74 million pet cats and their owners simply don't seem to count in the FDA/CVM's guardianship!

Are you mad yet? You should be. Because it didn't just magically end in 2002. Nothing changed because no one in authority seemed to care!

Petfoodindustry.com's April 2018 article states that the FDA did not initiate any new enforcement policies as a result of this study in 2002. So, for two decades, the industry has known of the problem, failed to supposedly locate it, and hence failed to resolve it. And yet we are made to believe that the FDA can track and trace to a single cow in 2003, when it was determined to have bovine spongiform encephalopathy (mad cow disease) in Washington state. The USDA set out and developed a national identification program by 2008-2009. That following year, APHIS (Animal and Plant Health Inspection Service) launched NAIS, a program between state and local government and the livestock industry to trace, manage and eradicate animal disease.

Well, first we need to learn what 4D meats or denatured meats are. "Denatured meat" is a meat product that has been processed specifically for the pet food market. This process is done to color the meat, showing it is no longer fit for human consumption. In the US, this product is then called "4D meat", and is once again regulated by the USDA. Other countries have other names for this process. This denaturing process involves making sure the "meat" cannot be rerouted back into the human food chain.

Meat from animals which are dead, diseased, disabled or dying (4-D meat) on arrival at the plant is most often salvaged for rendering, and then used by a wide range of industries, not limited to pet food manufacturers and zoos.

Rendering is a process that converts what is considered waste animal tissue, into a stable usable material. Rendering can also refer to any processing of animal products into more useful materials, such as the rendering of whole animal fatty tissue into purified fats like lard or tallow. Rendering by itself is not a bad plan and can be carried out on an industrial scale, farm level, or even in your own kitchen. When you take a cut of meat and trim it, that is a form of rendering. It can also be applied to non-animal products as well. But for our purposes of pet food and animal products, the majority of tissue processed comes from slaughterhouses. Also included, can be restaurant grease, butcher shop trimmings, and expired meat from grocery stores. This material can include the fatty tissue, bones, and also entire carcasses of animals condemned at slaughterhouses, and those that have died on farms or in transit, etc. The most common animal sources are beef, pork, mutton, and poultry.

The rendering process simultaneously dries the material and separates the fat from the bone and protein. This process yields a fat commodity (yellow grease, choice white grease, bleachable tallow, etc.)

and a protein meal powder (meat and bone meal, poultry byproduct meal, etc.) then sold to most any and all takers.

Okay, this all sounds good right? So, what are you talking about "pets eating pets" you crazy person? Well, it turns out that according to AAFCO, (remember Association of American Feed Control Officials?), pet food industry meat can come from virtually any mammal. So, generic meat meal produced from the rendering plants can be legally made from road kill, dead, diseased, or dying farm animals, and even euthanized cats and dogs. And there are still no laws or regulations forbidding the use of these euthanized pets in commercial pet food!

Sounds like a wild conspiracy theory, doesn't it? Well, around the year 1998, a brief news story was caught on tape from a Seattle news station KING of then President Hersch Pendell, of the Association of American Feed Control Officials, stating, "aesthetically it may not be acceptable, but nutritionally it's still protein". The interviewer then asks, "Can we tell what's in pet food just by looking at the label?" Pendell's response is, "There is no way to really tell that, because if the ingredients says 'meat and bone meal' you (meaning the consumer) don't know if that's cattle or sheep or a horse or fluffy".

Holy smokes, an admission from the industries number one (at the time) guy!

This book is hoping you will understand that processed rendered kibble is simply *not* the answer to feeding your kitty. But there is a whole rabbit hole of information out there if you wish to further your studies on this subject. Two of them are *Food Pets Die For* by Ann N Martin, and *Dead Pets Don't Lie* by Joe Ardis & Donna Howell. Our aim is to open your eyes to *why* you need to take these subjects seriously, and in Miss Kitty's best interest.

Here's how the circle can go. You purchase a sweet and adorable kitten along with a bag of kibble suggested by the nice veterinarian or pet food retailer. Miss Kitty grows up eating this kibble, but at three years of age gets a severe urinary tract infection. No big deal, everyone gets sick once in a while, right? Sure, of course. The kind well-meaning vet then prescribes a different diet, but again a processed kibble and Miss Kitty does well for a while. But then she develops crystals in her urine, causing her pain and discomfort. So, the well-intended veterinarian then prescribes yet a different type of diet, but again a processed kibble. Maybe this time with some of the same brand's canned offerings. And you go home thinking all will be well. Well around five or six, Miss Kitty now has a bloated belly, is considered extremely overweight, and maybe even diabetic. So, yup to the rescue is that same well-meaning vet, who again prescribes a new diet and now Miss Kitty is on insulin. So now you have not only a very expensive and potentially ineffective diet with an obese cat, but maybe even daily injections of insulin, which then require, often times weekly, monthly or bimonthly blood draws to make sure the insulin is working correctly. Now, a new problem to contend with is, injecting insulin into the same site day after day can also lead to the formation of a granuloma, or a lump of tissue. Or worse, the body may treat injectable insulin as a hostile intruder and form antibodies to attack the medication. Now you have an immune-compromised kitty that requires extreme and expensive care. *Maybe* this could have all been avoided if you had chosen to feed Miss Kitty the way Miss Kitty's DNA told her she should eat. At no point in time did Miss Kitty ever go out on those dry desert planes and say "Hey look! The elusive round red ball of crunchy hardened rendered grain product sprayed with fat to taste good! Let's catch it, kill it, and eat it." Everyone likes to eat at McDonald's from time to time, that's what treats are for. But day-to-day, Miss Kitty needs a healthy, easy-to-digest-for-her, piece of meat her body understands.

Or, look at this scenario again. You purchase a sweet and adorable kitten along with the obligatory bag of brightly colored kibble. Miss Kitty grows up, but at some point develops cancer. You cry and do the humane thing, and ask the local Animal Control or Humane Society to help you by euthanizing your sweet kitty. They follow through and offer you a beloved footprint in clay or other memory and you return home. Now the kitty is turned over to your local collection company they are contracted with who then in turn sells all those pets remains to a rendering plant. Remember, this is in no way illegal. So now your beloved pet, who had cancer, *and* was injected with a euthanasia solution, who maybe has a microchip embedded or even a collar on, is put into a huge vat with all the other meats, and "rendered" into the next batch of meat and bone meal powder sold to the next pet food manufacturer. Which then turns that meat and bone meal powder into the next bag of pet food found on your store shelves. And we wonder why cancer rates are potentially skyrocketing in our pets?

What ends up in the rendering plant's massive vats can be, not only your beloved pet, but also their collar, their microchip, their disease (cancers, puss, dirt from wounds, flies, maggots (remember road kill is picked up as well, that's the first part of the 4Ds) the plastic bag they are in or other covering if there is any, and for large livestock animals that may need to be mechanically hauled there, could be chain grease, dirt, gravel or pebbles.

Now as you can imagine, the pet food industry has denied all of the above for decades– but wait! Remember that interview from then President Hersch Pendell, of the Association of American Feed Control Officials? Hmmm... maybe he was mistaken? Or speaking out of turn? Doubtful.

Try watching the episode of "Dirty Jobs" with Mike Rowe entitled "Animal Rendering". This episode aired Jan 20, 2009 and clearly shows how meat, tissue and dead animals are processed and rendered, including the ambiguity of these terms.

Or how about, (found within the pages of this October 2017 *South Coast Air Quality Management District Rule Book*) the following:

> *It should be noted that 4 of the facilities render material from slaughter, meat packing, butcher shops, and grocery stores, one facility renders animals from zoos, euthanized animals from humane societies, and animals that are collected by counties and cities that died for various reasons. This rendering facility uses a batch-type cooking process.*

There it is in black and white. No big mystery is it? But the average person simply doesn't know. Or doesn't *want* to know it. It is no secret. Our lost, unwanted, unclaimed, old and debilitated pets get rendered into meat and bone meal powder that then gets sold to pet supply companies.

Okay, so that's a bit uncomfortable. That is a bit icky. So, Miss Kitty Number 1 can potentially end up feeding Miss Kitty Number 2!

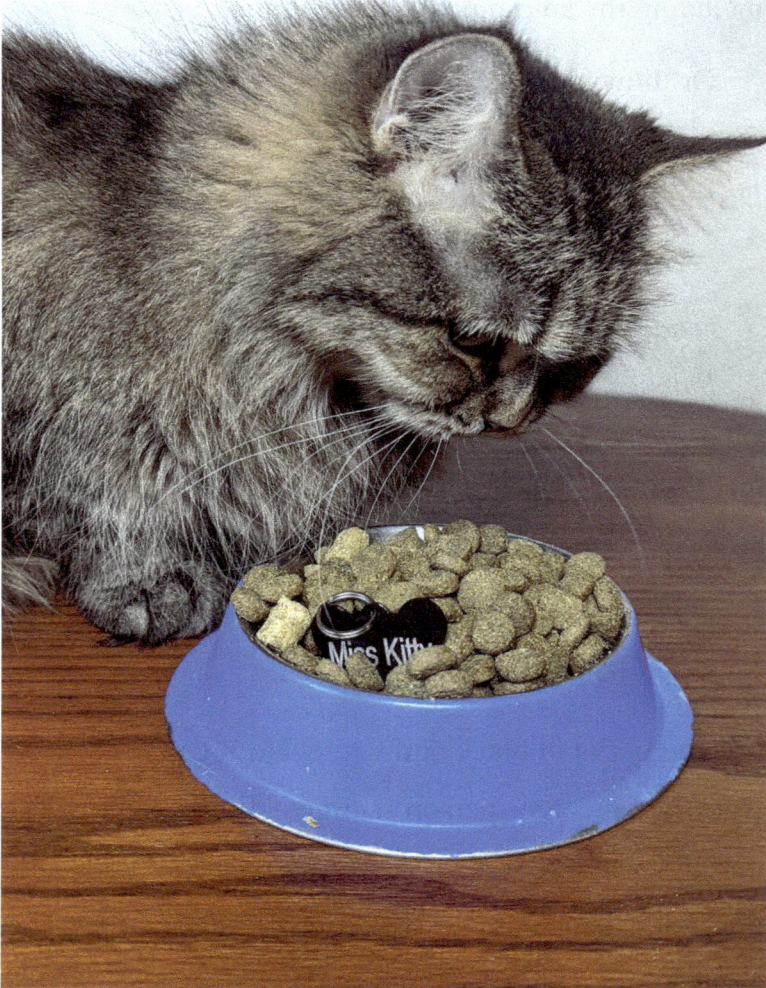

Chapter 7
Grains Give Me Tummy Pains

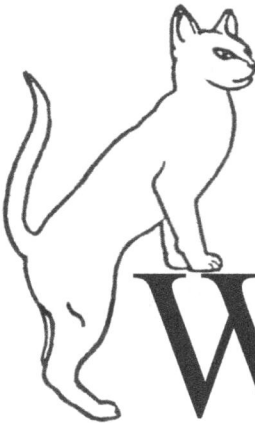

W e have already discussed and dissected that cats are obligate carnivores. This isn't a debate. So why do pet food companies and many vets treat them like small dogs, or worse– ruminants? We know protein is the basis for any feline's diet. So why do we as concerned, caring pet owners, continue to believe the crap-advertising these companies spew forth daily on our televisions and radios?

This is truly a situation of "not all things are created equal". Or maybe it would be better to say, "not all things are digested equally"! Most pet foods today contain some kind of grain, you just may not realize how much or what kind, and certainly not what quality.

Corn straight from the cob provides about 4 grams of protein for 1 cup, while an ear of corn weighing 3 ounces has about 3 grams of protein. One cup of prepared brown rice has about 5 grams of protein. The same amount of cooked couscous offers 6 grams, while a 1-cup portion of hot lentils is close to 18 grams of protein. Green peas have an even higher protein level at 8.25 grams of protein per cup, when boiled. A 1/4 cup of Lima beans has around 3.5 grams of protein. But they are all incomplete, each lacking in a few of the essential amino acids.

When a label reads as the one on the opposite page, you have to wonder if they remember they are feeding a cat? Were they mistaken on the type of carnivore? Did it ever cross their minds that this was not a biologically appropriate food, or that they could be causing grievous health issues when fed long-term? Nope, they see dollar signs. And still do today.

"Ground Yellow Corn, Corn Gluten Meal, Chicken By-Product Meal, Soybean Meal, Beef Tallow (Preserved with Mixed Tocopherols), Animal Digest, Calcium Carbonate, Turkey By-Product Meal, Salmon Meal, Ocean Fish Meal, Phosphoric Acid, Choline Chloride, Salt, Potassium Chloride, Titanium Dioxide (Color), Vitamins [Vitamin E Supplement, Niacin Supplement, Vitamin A Supplement, D-Calcium Pantothenate, Thiamine Mononitrate (Source of Vitamin B1), Riboflavin Supplement (Source of Vitamin B2), Pyridoxine Hydrochloride (Source of Vitamin B6), Menadione Sodium Bisulfite Complex (Source of Vitamin K Activity), Vitamin D3 Supplement, Folic Acid, Biotin, Vitamin B12 Supplement], Minerals [Ferrous Sulfate (Source of Iron), Zinc Oxide, Manganous Oxide, Copper Sulfate, Calcium Iodate, Sodium Selenite], Taurine, Yellow 6, Yellow 5, Red 40, Blue 2, Rosemary Extract."

Now this is where it gets "fun". (Or at least educational, I hope.) This product claims it is "100% Complete and Balanced Nutrition". It claims it has "high quality protein", and also claims to have a whopping 30% protein! How can that be, when the first ingredient is ground yellow corn and the second ingredient is corn gluten meal? Remember, just because there is protein in a food, doesn't mean it is "bioavailable". There's that pesky word again.

So, let's learn to read those labels– what they are really saying and why. Again, it is oh so important. Here's a quick tip– it's all in the wording. How they say these things is exceptionally important. Little wording differences can and do make huge differences in the actual content of the product. Some examples include:

1. Chicken (insert any protein here) Food for cats

2. Chicken Dinner or Chicken Recipe

3. Cat Food with Chicken

4. Chicken Flavored Cat Food, or Cat Food Flavored with Chicken.

Let's take these one by one individually...

#1 – The protein of your choice food for cats. This falls under the AAFCO 95% rule and would indicate that this product is required to have at least 95% of the specified protein, not counting water weight (more on this shortly).

#2 – This is more than a change in the language, it means it has less of the specified protein, much less. Foods with this designation need to only have "at least" 25% of the named protein.

#3 – This contains even less of the specified protein, and must only contain no less than 3% of the named protein in question. Makes you wonder what the remaining 97% of the ingredients are?

And then there is the lowest of the low...

#4 – "Flavored". As in, there is some specified protein, but tests haven't really picked up a specific amount. Really? Testing can't even detect an amount? Holy scam Batman!

AAFCO model regulations specify the exact wording of the product names according to how much of the animal-based ingredients the food actually contains.

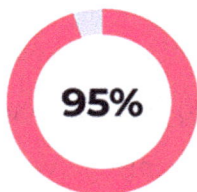

95% — If it contains 95% meat labels will read: *Beef Dog Food, Chicken Dog Food, etc.*

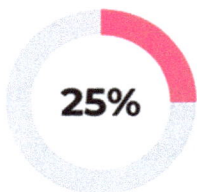

25% — If it contains a minimum of 25% meat labels will read: *Chicken Dinner, Recipe or Entree, etc.*

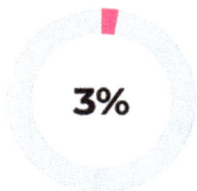

3% — If it contains only 3% meat labels will read: "With", "Contains" Beef, Chicken, etc.

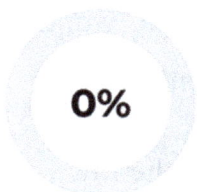

0% — If it contains only trace amounts labels will read: *Chicken Flavor!, Flavoring, etc.*

Always make sure to consider the way an ingredient list can split ingredients. Think of corn. Some ingredient labels will list flaked corn, ground corn, and kibbled corn, which adds up to a lot of corn! Yet without a careful reading of the ingredient label, you may not realize how much corn is in the food.

Let's use this as an example:

You are starving, and all there is to eat are bricks. Cool! Bricks contain calcium, phosphorous, potassium, and sodium, so they must be healthy right? Go ahead, take a bite, chew it up and swallow. A little dry right? And all those great minerals are inaccessible to our craving bodies, because we don't have a digestive tract made to break this particular item down. So, what happens? We are quite literally "shitting bricks" and still starving to death. But it's all we have, so we eat more.

Getting the picture yet?

Miss Kitty is hungry; her body is telling her she needs to eat to fuel her activities and stay healthy, but all she has is an extruded, processed, high heat-cooked piece of meal that is mostly corn, wheat or soy! But she is hungry so she eats. And we have been taught that corn is an excellent source of protein, carbohydrates, and fiber. Too bad she does not have a digestive tract capable of breaking down this cooked salad nugget mess. So, what happens? She is quite literally "crapping corn" back into the litterbox. But she's still hungry, so she eats more of the high-heat-cooked, extruded piece of meal, because she relies on us to serve her needs. And we failed her. Not intentionally, but to her detriment, nonetheless.

79

A quick note about *Ash*...

On the back of a lot of cat food products, even today is this thing called "Ash". But what is it and why do we care? Pretty simply, ash is just the burnt remains when the food you are looking at gets incinerated (at a higher than 500° F temperature). These inorganic materials, the minerals can be any combination of calcium, magnesium, phosphorus, potassium, sodium, silicon, sulfur and other trace minerals.

In the 70s and 80s, most vets were blaming this ash content for the crystals in the urine and especially the boy cats for "blocking", which is a life-threatening situation. However, additional research and increased knowledge has now shown that the main problem was the formulation of commercial pet foods. Pet foods were creating a more alkaline urine (higher pH) which led to an increase in struvite (magnesium ammonium phosphate) crystals. Commercial dry kibble diets are almost always formulated with a high vegetable and grain content. This creates a more alkaline urine, generally higher than 7.0. A high-meat, natural raw cat food diet, such as a cat would eat in nature creates a more acidic urine. Generally speaking, a cat's urine PH should be in the 6.0 -6.4 range. Remember, a lower number is higher acidity and better, generally speaking, for our Miss Kitty.

Chapter 8
Fear Mongering

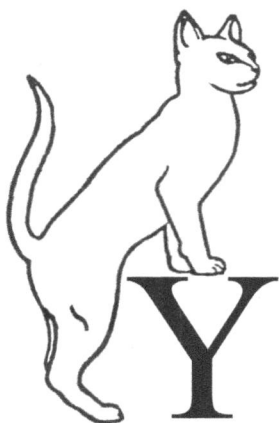

Y ou have read enough to know that you should be feeding Miss Kitty raw, but *EEK*! You've read up about it online, and "everyone" says how you will get Salmonella and die! Well okay, that's a bit of an exaggeration. Maybe not *everyone* is saying that, and maybe you won't die, but you'll be super sick for a super long time, and your whole family will be at risk, and you could kill Grandma! Okay, okay, calm down. Now that you have been thoroughly traumatized by all the horror stories and fear mongering, how about "let's talk turkey"...

Feeding a biologically appropriate diet to your pets is the most humane and logical thing you could do. Just like when we humans choose a salad over McDonalds.

One of the main sources of concern as well as the top tactic used to scare you into continuing your kibble barrage, is the fear of Salmonella. And it's a very valid fear. Salmonella is a type of bacteria that affects the intestinal tract of pets and people, and is typically spread and shed through feces. Yup – poop! According to the CDC, they estimate that each year in the US, approximately 1.35 million people become infected and affected, resulting in over 26,000 hospitalizations and as many as 420 deaths. Scary stuff, I know. And the main way humans contract Salmonella is through eating infected food.

Remember the great Romaine lettuce recall of 2020? How about the recent onion recall in 32 states in 2021? Isn't it great our food chain is so safe? No one seems to be saying, "Let's change our model of eating because some food sources have the slight potential for contamination." What they do is resolve those obvious problems, and notify the public when there is cause for concern to a large enough degree. And that's a good thing for everyone.

If you read the FDA's list of causes or exposures, there pretty much isn't anything safe from this little bugger of a bacteria. Your fish, your pet lizard, your lettuce, onions, eggs, dairy products, raw meat, poultry products, unpasteurized milk, and this list goes on. The FDA is even kind enough to warn us that our dogs and cats can be unaffected carriers and spread the bacterium throughout the house in the form of doggie kisses, cleaning of litter boxes, or of having stool (yup poop again) accidents where humans have to clean it up. Even horses can get this nasty little bugger as well, and share and spread it.

So, the dire warnings that we are all going to die if we feed our cats raw seems to be a bit premature. I honestly can't say that I have ever seen a cat catch their dinner then stop and knock on my door and say, "Hey bub, mind throwing this in the microwave for a few minutes?" Have you?

What you have to remember, is that the cat has a shortened digestive tract to specifically deal with these kinds of pathogens. Do some cats contract Salmonella? Clearly the answer is "yes". But I would ask, "What was their primary diet? Were they optimally healthy animals eating an optimal diet? Or were they already kibble-fed, dehydrated, obese, or diabetic?"

A healthy animal when fed properly, tends to *stay* healthy. Remember sixth grade science class and homeostasis? Same concept. Something else to keep in mind is that there are no vegan cats. It's simply not biologically possible, and could be construed as abuse.

"Great", you cry! "But what about me, my infant, and my aging grandmother? I surely don't want to risk them simply to feed my cat a biologically-appropriate diet." Well, have they contracted Salmonella thus far in their existence? "Of course not", you respond. "I know how to safely handle, prepare, and cook my meats." Well awesome, you just answered your own question. Safe and sanitary measures should always be used to make your cats new homemade raw diet. It's the same exact principals. Wash your counters with soap and water, and a disinfecting solution. Always use a cutting board. Always wash and disinfect the cutting board after each use. Always wash and disinfect your hands, both before and after preparing raw meats of any kind. Always keep meat, poultry, and eggs refrigerated, as well as refrigerating promptly or freezing when done. You can even go so far as to use a disposable paper plate if you don't wish to have raw meats touching your own personal plates.

Also, disposable gloves can be worn, and should be by pregnant women and those who are immunocompromised, immunosuppressed, or believe themselves to be.

Another in a long line of arguments against feeding your Miss Kitty correctly, is money. The battle cry here is "but it's SOOO expensive". Um, that just doesn't hold water.

Here's some really good basic math for you, from Maine Coon Breeder Glen Siegel from a January 2022 social media post:

"We made 80 lbs of raw cat food today at a cost of $225 which is $2.81 a lbs below is what's in it. Just to compare this batch with a popular canned food, lets pick Purina cat food (not my favorite but something people use) Purina cost $35 for 24 5.5 oz cans.

The math:

24 x 5.5 oz. = 132 oz.
132 oz. / 16 oz in a lb. = 8.25 lb.
$35 / 8.25 lb. = $4.24 a lb.

What's in our raw from the supermarket:

14.5 lb. Cornish Game Hen Whole
1-1 lb. Chicken Heart
7 lb. Chicken Thigh with bone
5 lb. Chicken Liver
20 lb. Chicken Breast boneless
2 lb. Beef Kidney
5 lb. Salmon
32 Eggs
2 lb. Pumpkin
4 Quarts Water
4 lb. Sardines
20 Teaspoon Kittybloom VM 900+3
16 Teaspoons Super Lysine

3 hours from start to finish.

Now read what's in any other canned cat food."

This is a great narrative to show how making your own is not only healthier for Miss Kitty, but your wallet as well. Clearly, this recipe makes a lot of food, and that is definitely a great choice if you have a lot of room in your freezer and/or a lot of cats to feed. But for most folks with one, two, or three kitties, this might not be the most practical.

So, use a calculator and cut the recipe in half to start. Look at the numbers and see if this is still too large a portion for you to be comfortable with. If not, cut in half again. See how simple that was?

Chapter 9
Let's Get
Started

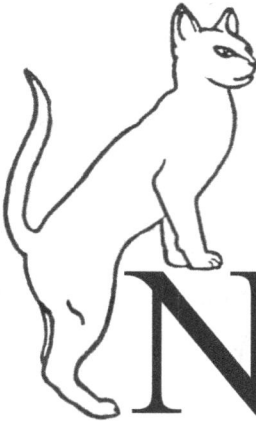

Now you know why you should be feeding raw to your kitty. Now you know why you shouldn't be feeding processed, cooked kibble. Now you know why your kitty's health could be suffering from the use of the processed cooked kibble, and you want to do better. Congratulations!

But there are still some generalities you should be aware of before beginning to make your own diets. Not everything is cut and dried. Be flexible. This is a biggie! Your kitty eats what you give them, day in and day out.

It is once again, up to you to make meals more than a boring "Ground Hog Day" repetition of the same ole thing. And realize, this is a quick generalization of foods, and not to be considered a complete breakdown of individual items. Use common sense. Research from reliable sources who have had success feeding raw diets, and find out what works best for your Miss Kitty.

Chicken is an easy, cost-effective meat that is easy to source for most. And many, if not most, raw food recipes are written with chicken as the base meat used. However, factory-farmed chicken can be highly inflammatory, and even with the addition of omega-3s, it is very difficult to balance the omega-6 levels in chicken. Rotation is important for so many reasons!

And speaking of rotations, cats are generalist carnivores, which means that they eat a wide variety of prey animals that are available in their environment – not just one kind. They don't look at that sparrow and think, "Nope, I only eat pigeon". They don't look at the mouse and go, "Nope, you are over 6-months-old, think I'll pass". Cats are true hunters and eat all prey animals in their territory.

Turkey is another great source of easy-to-use, easy-to-find in your local market protein source. Be sure to read the labeling, because more often than not, as much as 15% "broth" has been added, and that often times not only contains salts, but nitrates and unknown (unlabeled) spices. Turkey often has rosemary and other "natural flavors" added.

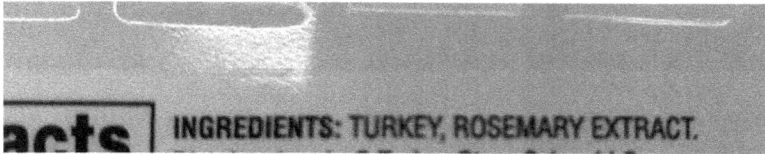

INGREDIENTS: TURKEY, ROSEMARY EXTRACT.

You want the sodium to be under 100mg per serving (4 oz). Turkey as well as chicken, is often easier to cut with meat preparation scissors when still partially frozen to "chunk" it.

Pork is a great meat to include in your cat's raw diet, as it is an excellent source of thiamine. Many cats really like pork, and again it can be a cost effective easily-sourced food. Farmed pork in most countries, including the US and Canada, as well as many EU countries, is perfectly safe to feed. However, wild boar, Javelina, etc. should not be fed raw due to concerns with pseudorabies.

Bones. Make no bones about it, bones are excellent for kitties, even those not on a raw diet. Especially for those not on an all-raw diet! They are great teeth-cleaners. They work the jaw muscles. Raw bones are soft and pliable and do not splinter. Miss Kitty-sized bones include chicken wings, rabbit ribs, chicken necks (sparingly), whole prey, even chicken feet with the nails clipped off. Raw chicken necks are an amazing source of nutrition, exercise, and mental satisfaction to a cat, but need to be given sparingly– no more than 1 or 2 times a week at most. Necks can still have bits of thyroid tissue clinging to the meat. This source of thyroid is a natural source of iodine and could be a contributing factor of hyperthyroidism that is common in cats. Again, we highly argue for rotation and variety. Bones also add additional calcium and can unbalance the ratio if given on a too-frequent basis. And of course, common sense says you should always supervise your cat when giving raw bones to make sure they don't have any problems with them. Bone content in most homemade diets, and even pre-made diets is almost always felt to be 80% meat to 10% bone to 10% liver/organs. (80/10/10). Birds and small rodents however, are generally more along the lines of between 4-8% bone, so your diet make-up should take this into account. Too much bone can lead to constipation, and too high a calcium content. Remember cats are not small dogs.

When speaking of calcium, many folks use egg shell to supplement. Eggs are a superior source of nutrition, including protein, Vitamin A, biotin, selenium, iron, riboflavin, and other essential fatty acids. Just remember that egg shell is not a supplement for bone.

Thiamine, also known as B1, is essential for all living creatures, including our Miss Kitty. Great sources of it include pork as already discussed, and small oily fish such as anchovies or sardines. You will find that generally a diet too high in fish is a bad idea and leads to many nutritive deficiencies, however adding in just a bit for variety and rotation can be a great source of pleasure and nutrition for your kitty. And the bones of the fish are almost entirely digestible and bioavailable!

Thiamine deficiencies are rampant in the packaged processed food industry. In 2017 AVA brand of dry kibble was recalled for this very problem in the UK,

THE RAW FACTS OF FELINE FEEDING

and many cats were adversely affected. Some euthanized before and after the recall. For a simple vitamin deficiency! It's horrifying.

Eggs are nature's greatest food – 98% digestible. Feeding whole eggs, including the shell and yolks raw are an amazing and important source for any raw diet. It is not advised to feed the whites individually, as these can lead to deficiencies. There is a protein in the egg whites, that can bind to certain B-specific vitamins, preventing them from being absorbed and available.

Rotating proteins and base mix, as well as completers and vitamins, helps keep things fresh and exciting for Miss Kitty. Just some of the protein sources out there commercially available are:

- Chicken
- Turkey
- Pork
- Beef
- Bison
- Elk/Deer
- Emu/Ostrich
- Goat
- Sheep/Lamb
- Farmed Fish
- Pheasant/Quail
- Squab
- Duck/Geese
- Rabbit

And I am sure I am missing some. Frozen, you can purchase rats, mice, day-old quail/chicks (DOQ), gerbils, hamsters, and a few others.

Something that gets overlooked is the house cricket. This is a great source of hunting prey/play experience for Miss Kitty, and a clean source of prey that won't have most folks following behind with a spray bottle and sanitizer. Crickets can be bought at most pet shops, and PetCo® stores throughout the US. One thing to caution is being wary of "wild" crickets – that could have mites or pesticides sprayed on them.

Taurine is another of those life-giving essentials to cats, that they can only get through their food. A deficiency in taurine will lead to feline retinal degeneration and blindness, dilated cardiomyopathy, and eventually heart failure which in turn will result in the cat's death. This is not something to mess around with. Other disorders such as an inadequate immune response (meaning your cat is chronically ill), poor neonatal growth, poor reproduction and congenital defects are also on the hit parade of taurine deficiency. And by feeding a raw diet, (if making it yourself), it must be done right, so as to prevent any of the above from occurring. And here's the great thing about taurine– If you do "overdo" it a bit from time to time, no worries. Miss Kitty will just excrete it out in her litter box when she pees. Now, taurine can be affected by a number of factors, rendering it less bioavailable. Things such as heat processing, as well as certain fibers which bind to taurine, which are found in lower-quality foods, (particularly rice bran) can all contribute to whatever taurine is found in the food, being unusable to Miss Kitty.

Note that until the end of the 1980s, it wasn't known that additional taurine was needed in processed cat food, and so taurine wasn't added to commercial cat food such as kibble or canned. One of the main causes of death for cats during that time was dilated cardiomyopathy, unknowingly caused by taurine deficiency. Once discovered, companies started supplementing this essential nutrient, but not until pet owners got involved and studies were done.

The general NRC guideline for adult cats is a recommendation of 250 mg per 1000 kcal. The great thing is, taurine is found in virtually all meat sources to some degree, and raw diets often don't need too much additional supplementation. Chicken thighs are higher in taurine than chicken breasts, and chicken hearts are higher still.

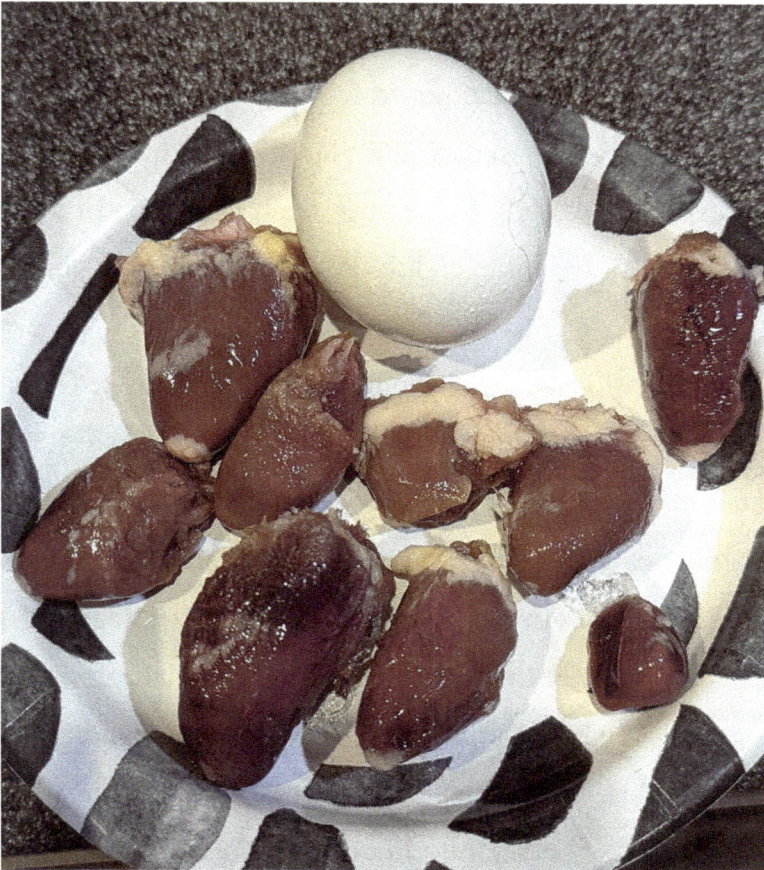

Knowing where to look for taurine is important to the goal of making your own foods. Found almost exclusively in animal products, it's in the highest concentration in seafoods, hard-working muscles like the heart and tongue, and poultry dark meat (meat from the thigh). Smaller animals are richer in taurine than larger animals, while whole prey such as mice, rats, day-old chicks and quail, are quite rich in taurine. Then you have those foods that are quite low on the taurine scale such as rabbit, chicken breasts, and any meats that have been mechanically deboned (processed). Remember, fresh is best, and variety is not only the spice of life, but can be the key to not running into long-term deficiencies.

The basic take-away should be that you can feed most any meats that you think your cat will like. The exception being that you don't want to feed other carnivores. Fish should not be used as a main protein, and wild boar should not be fed raw. Any wild game should be frozen for at least three weeks prior to feeding, to kill any potential parasites.

One topic that is not often covered is that with Miss Kitty getting a raw diet, you may see her drinking less. While this is perfectly normal, you do still need to be aware of how much moisture she is getting.

Again, cats are desert dwellers by nature, and therefore designed to get their water from their food source. If in doubt, you can always add more moisture to your mix in the form of water, or even a good homemade bone broth.

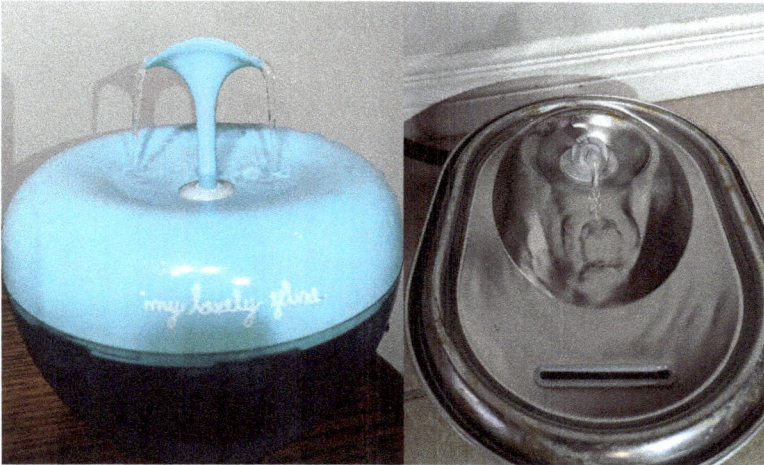

Note: You should not use most commercially available bone broths, as they contain much higher salt contents than is advisable, as well as ingredients that can harm your cat like onions and celery. Even those made for dogs often contain such unsuitable ingredients for cats.

There are multiple brands of completers for raw diets as well as a few complete vitamin mixes (essentially the same thing, just not labeled as such). Again, variety is the spice of life, and what one completer may have in abundance, another may not. If you have a kitty with health concerns such as kidney disease or ongoing IBD, be sure to do your research to find the ones that work best for your individual circumstances. Finding a holistic vet to support you in your journey is an invaluable asset for you. A few meal completers/complete vitamins are:

- ✤ **NuVet**, found at: https://www.nuvet.com/
  Be careful, there are many knock-offs with similar names.

- ✤ **EZ Complete Fur Cats**, found at:
  https://www.foodfurlife.com
  They offer 2 different size packages depending on your needs.

- ✤ **TCFeline** found at: https://tcfeline.com/tcfeline-premix/

- ✤ **Alnutrin** found at: https://www.knowwhatyoufeed.com/
  Offers several different varieties meeting different needs, including AAFCO certifications on some, and as a bonus they offer sample sizes to try!

- ✤ **Felini Complete** and **Felini Renal** (UK) found at:
  https://www.zooplus.com/

- ✤ **Raw Meow Mix** (AUS) found at:
  https://rawmeow.com.au/collections/raw-meow-mix

One thing to keep in mind, once you have completely transitioned over to a raw diet, is that you will notice a couple of things. You should notice that Miss Kitty's stool (yup her poop) will be overall less smelly, smaller in size, and less frequent. Stool is a really good indicator of overall health and the body's functions.

Also, you may notice less water intake. Now that Miss Kitty is eating a species-appropriate diet, much of her moisture needs should be being met by the raw diet you are feeding her. You can also add water to your fed-diet as well. Remember, we learned in Chapter 1 about not only structurally why, but evolutionarily why, cats are not well-suited to drinking large amounts of water. You must still always have fresh water available around the house, especially for those who don't have a Miss Kitty but rather a Mister Kitty. This helps ensure there is no reason for him to be dehydrated, potentially leading to a urinary tract blockage due to crystal formation.

Two words that are often used interchangeably are "balanced and complete". Do not make the mistake that they mean the same thing, for they most certainly do not. When we say that a raw food is "balanced", this typically refers to the meat/bone/organ ratio. And balanced can mean different things to different folks.

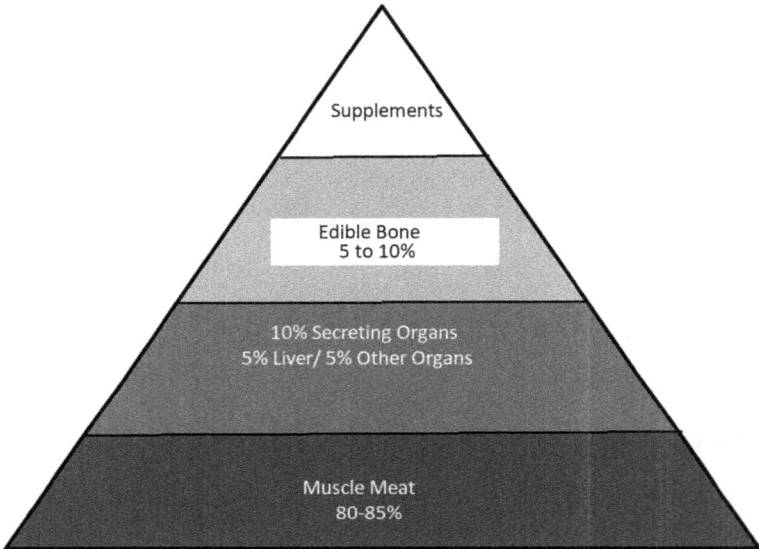

Commercially-prepared raw foods are often balanced to a ratio of 80/10/10. Prey Model Raw diets will more often use a ratio of 84/6/10. And many other types of food sold as raw cat food is neither complete nor balanced. So once again, it is completely up to the consumer to read and understand the labeling. Using a broad range and diversity of ingredients can help to balance these ratios out over time.

Now remember, these types of diets are not in any way complete. They still need the appropriate nutrients of vitamins and minerals to be added in.

One really good resource available online is a calculator for balancing these items. This calculator is very handy to know how much of each while keeping the overall ratio balanced:

http://www.rawcalc.org/dilute-bone-content.html

Watching your minimums and maximums of both vitamins and minerals is crucial as well. Fat-soluble vitamins should never exceed maximums, such as Vitamin E. These end up being stored in the fat rather than excreted.

"Complete" on the other hand, as we already know from previous chapters, refers to the food meeting the minimums or recommended daily allowances that were set by AAFC or NRC. These foods when labeled as such, already have vitamins and minerals added into their pre-made mix, and you should be extremely cautious when adding in more, or changing the food in any way.

Introducing New Food Chart

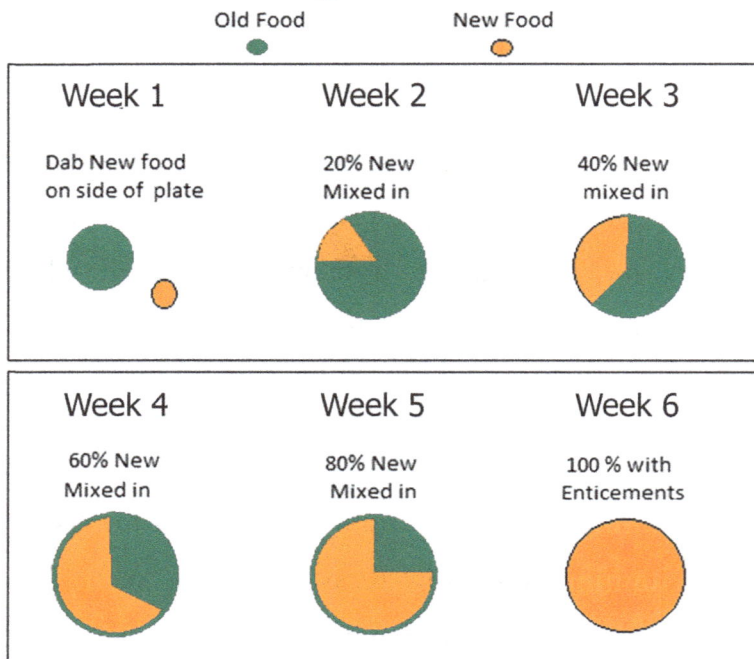

Old Food ●   New Food ○

Week 1	Week 2	Week 3
Dab New food on side of plate	20% New Mixed in	40% New mixed in

Week 4	Week 5	Week 6
60% New Mixed in	80% New Mixed in	100 % with Enticements

Getting started can take days or even weeks, depending on how well Miss Kitty receives her new and improved diet. Time and patience are needed, especially if your kitty is an adult already. Remember, she didn't become a McDonald's addict overnight, so she's not going to kick her habit overnight either.

The best time to start this endeavor is first thing in the morning. Pick up all her kibble and literally remove it from the house. Cats have a very good sense of smell. Here is where things can be a bit confusing for you.

We do advocate for multiple proteins rotated regularly, but when starting out, it is best to stick with the primary protein source that she is used to from her kibble. Start small. If it takes 3 days, then it takes 3 days. If it takes longer, then it takes longer. For adult cats, you may see some loose stools when first introducing raw meat diets until their digestive tract adjusts. Often adding a bit of digestive aid powder such as Forti Flora or S Boulardii can help ease this transition time.

Often times, if you have a cat who has been fed kibble her whole life, it can be easier to transition with a "gateway" high-quality canned food. One that follows the same principals using no grains, peas or legumes. Jarred meat baby foods can be used as an enticement as well. Read your labels carefully. Generally, we only recommend Gerber® brand Stage 2 strained meats at this time for this purpose.

Freeze-dried raw hearts and livers crumbled up can be added to entice a reluctant eater as well. And even catnip can be sprinkled lightly into a new diet to entice that most picky of eaters. Remember to remove the dry food from the house. Cats smell almost as well as dogs, you aren't fooling anyone by putting that bag of yummy pretty extruded colorized crap in a high cupboard.

Time and patience are key. Never let a cat starve past 24 hours.

Enticements can be many things. A small portion of bonito flakes can kick-start Miss Kitty to eating. Use a plate or saucer, not a bowl. Act as if the food is yours and "protect" it from Miss Kitty.

You can even go so far as to "drop" a bit of it. Nothing is better than stolen goodies!

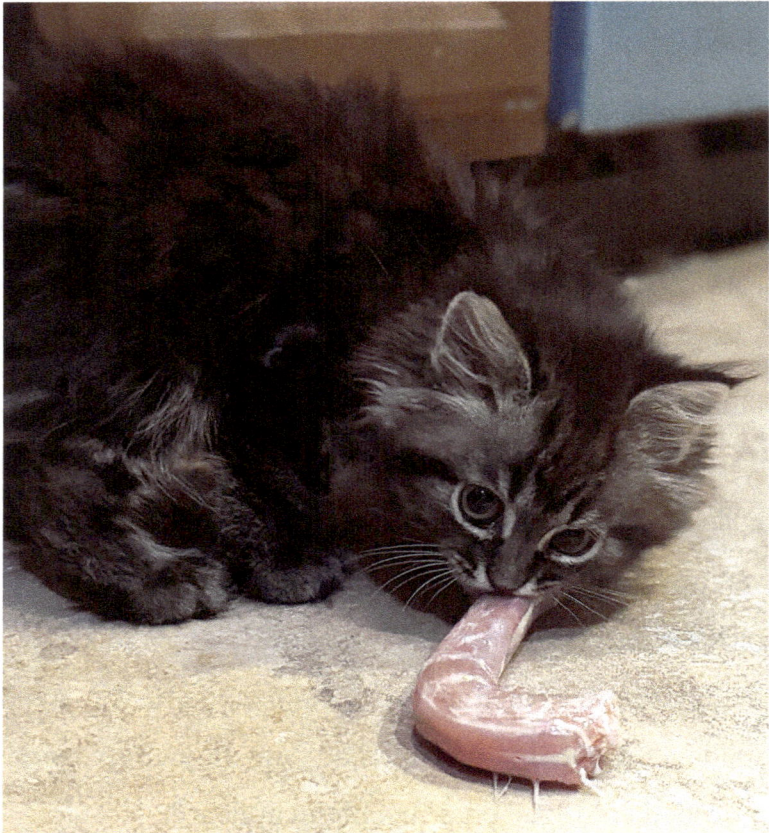

Chapter 10
The Skinny on Raw Diets

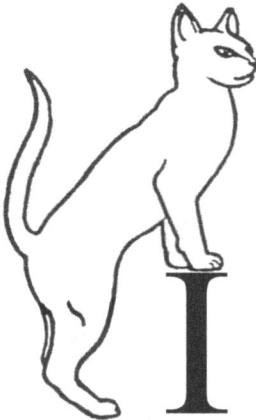

I take it because you have read this far, you are ready to make the proverbial leap and start feeding your little obligate carnivore like a feline, and no longer like any other type of creature on this big diverse planet. Awesome, I applaud you. And Miss Kitty thanks you too. But now what? What's your next step?

First you need to recognize what you can do and how far you are willing to work at this. Raw diets are produced both commercially or at home. How much time you can devote, is entirely up to you. Commercial, as discussed, come with a much higher cost per serving ratio, shipping issues, and the potential for your kitty to turn their nose up at it once you've invested quite a bit into it.

At the end of this book is a partial list of readily available commercially prepared raw frozen and freeze-dried raw diets. This is by no means a complete list, nor are we endorsing any one over any other. It is there for your convenience and to be able to give you a starting point.

The next type of diets are the basic starters. These are raw meat, again commercially prepared, but they are *not* complete diets. These will still require you to add a vitamin/meat completer to the diet along with some water and sometimes even some oils or eggs.

Read the labels carefully, and be sure to know which ones need which ingredients. These can be a little cheaper, as they aren't the complete product. However, you incur more expense by still buying and storing several other additional ingredients. Although, these have the really great option of being able to be changed-out in many different ways. For instance, one week you can prepare a starter meat – let's use a ground chicken, hearts, liver, and bone mix, and you want to add your completer mix as well as some tripe. "Viola!" Then next week, you decide to change things up a bit, and add some nice ground lamb you got on sale as well as the vitamin completer. But this time Miss Kitty decides to turn her nose up at this particular addition. Perfectly simple, and you are not stuck with a huge batch. You have a few days' worth that you may be able to mix into something else that she *does* care for later. Don't be afraid to try out new proteins and organs, and even use more than one completer. Keeping Miss Kitty engaged in her meals, and not becoming married to one sole source of protein (taste) or completer (texture) will only benefit you both in the long run.

Next, we have the Whole Prey Model (WPM) type of diets, and they are probably the most controversial and rarest. Yup, it is exactly as it sounds. Whole animals, such as small rats, mice, baby quail, and baby chicks to name a few. These are particularly fun for Miss Kitty, as they can not only keep her healthy, but provide mental stimulation as well. Believe it or not, cats get mental satisfaction in doing the tasks they were designed to do. This active engagement in their meal has many positive benefits. Tearing, ripping and scissoring through meat, tendons and bones provides the necessary stimulation to keep your carnivore's mouth clean and healthy, their mind active and engaged, and their gut in sync with the rest of the body. Feeding a Prey Model type of diet means much less preparation time and less overall work, with minimal or even no supplementation. Whole prey is probably the rarest of the feeding models because most folks find it distasteful to see one animal eat another.

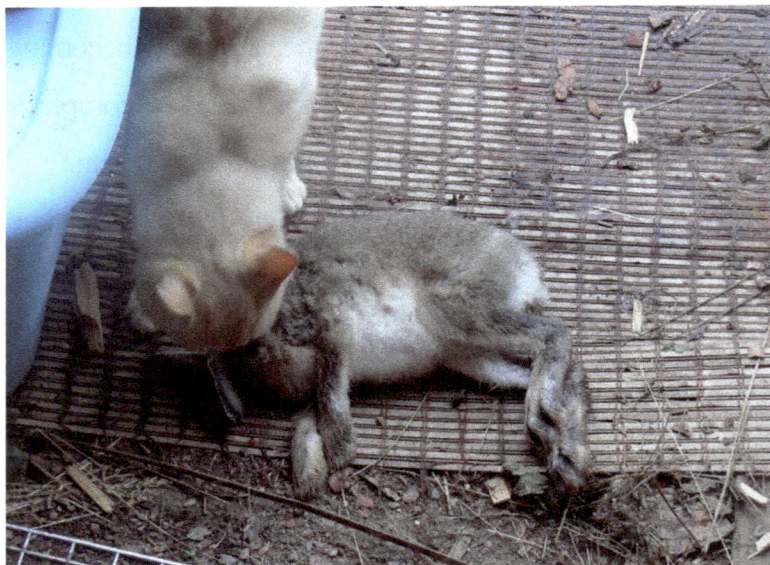

We have been so removed from the natural food chain ourselves that mentally, many just can't do it. And that's fine, there are many other options.

Some cats can't even recognize whole prey if they've been fed a lifetime of processed kibble, and may need to be slowly adjusted into in using other methods first.

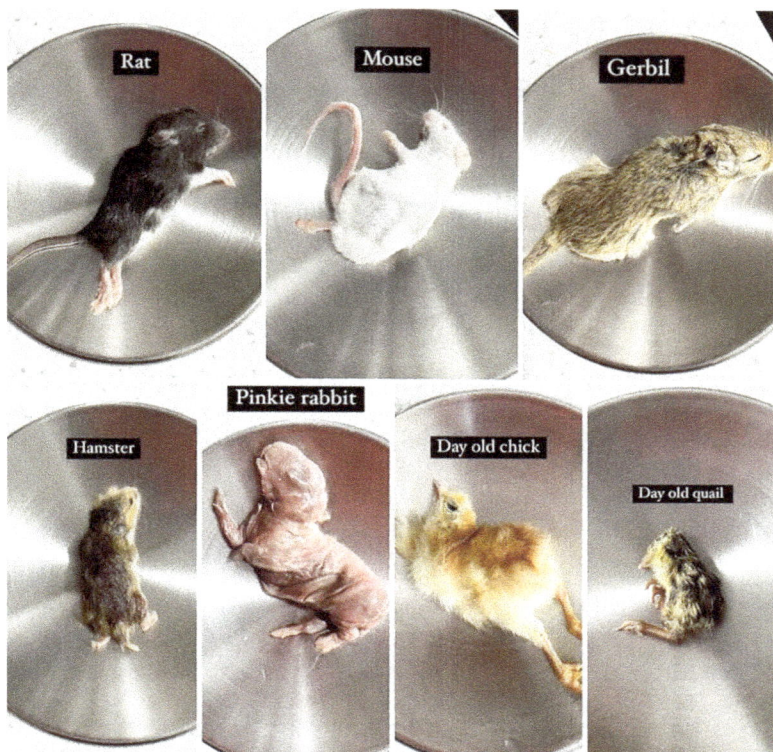

Also, there is a similar method to Whole Prey, generally called Prey Model Raw, which is building a recipe to mimic the above-mentioned Whole Prey. Using this method still adheres to the general principal of 80/10/5/5 (or 80/6ish/5ish/5ish for using secreting organs) and requires the added small oily fish, eggs, kelp, other organ parts, and some supplements. This method generally requires much more time and money, and is harder to maintain long-term, which runs the risk of Miss Kitty missing out on key nutrients.

Finally, we have the make-it-yourself-from-scratch raw diet. This is by far the most popular type of raw feeding, and also the easiest to make many mistakes, with potentially allowing Miss Kitty to be nutrient-deficient over time. You must make the commitment to this type of feeding. It takes time to source all of the ingredients, and it takes time and care to learn the recipes that work from many different sources. Making the diet can be time-consuming as well.

It is immensely satisfying to make your cat's meals, knowing what goes into it and more importantly knowing what is *not* in it. But it is not a simple matter. You have to purchase the preparatory items and make sure your workspace is free of distractions. You don't need the kids running in and setting their Gameboys down on the counter that just had fresh chicken on it!

Like the other diets, you will have to learn more than one recipe, because you will be changing it up from time to time. Often times, this is where being in a larger group of like-minded people can really help you out. Online social groups often have a "group think" kind of atmosphere and can help you out with all kinds of answers, tips, tricks and options you may not have even known existed! I highly suggest you find a group or two, join up and lurk for a while. See if that group fits your needs, and fits your beliefs of how to feed Miss Kitty. If not, go ahead and find another one, there are plenty out there. But always remember that making a mistake in one or two meals is not the end of the world. Learn, try again and you *will* do better next time!

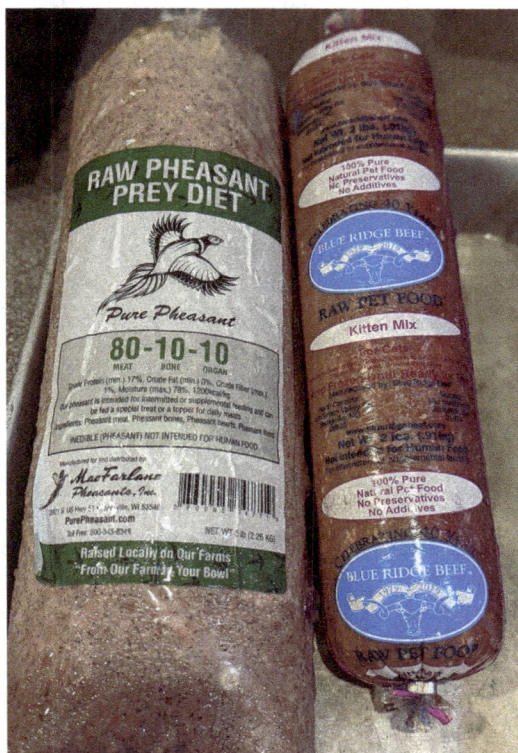

Don't Be Fooled!

Here's a word of warning to the wise, and you are certainly now wiser than you were before! You know those fancy labels that say "organic", and cost a larger fortune? Do not be suckered in by them. There are zero, that's right *zero* regulations currently at the time of this writing for organic pet foods.

In 2004, the National Organic Program decided to create a task force "to develop labeling standards for organic pet food".

"The National Organic Standards Board (NOSB) at its October 12-14, 2004, meeting recommended the formation of two ad hoc task force groups to develop draft organic standards. One task force will develop proposed production, handling, and labeling standards for food and animal feed products derived from aquatic animals. The second task force will develop proposed organic labeling standards for pet food."

Wait, what? Not one but two task forces? Yup, and since 2004. And then like all good government bodies it took them 4 years to release their "recommendations", which at that time included definitions of organic along with labeling requirements. Then, in 2010 the AAFCO website posted an "Update on Organic Pet Foods", but here's the exciting part, (well for the industry at least), instead of releasing guidelines as previously submitted, the update was from the pet food industry itself! (The Pet Food Institute.) Remember early-on how the pet food industry got to set their own nutritional values? Yeah, it's kind of like that.

So, we have the existing organic laws which don't mention pet food at all, and basically, they are free to interpret them any way they want. And believe me, they do.

Without specific organic pet food regulations, regulatory authorities in the pet food industry have nothing to enforce, should the regulatory authority disagree with a manufacturer's interpretation of the law.

Remember how the alphabet soup of government agencies "oversee" the pet food industry as it is, and that the new National Organic Program falls under the jurisdiction of the USDA as well.

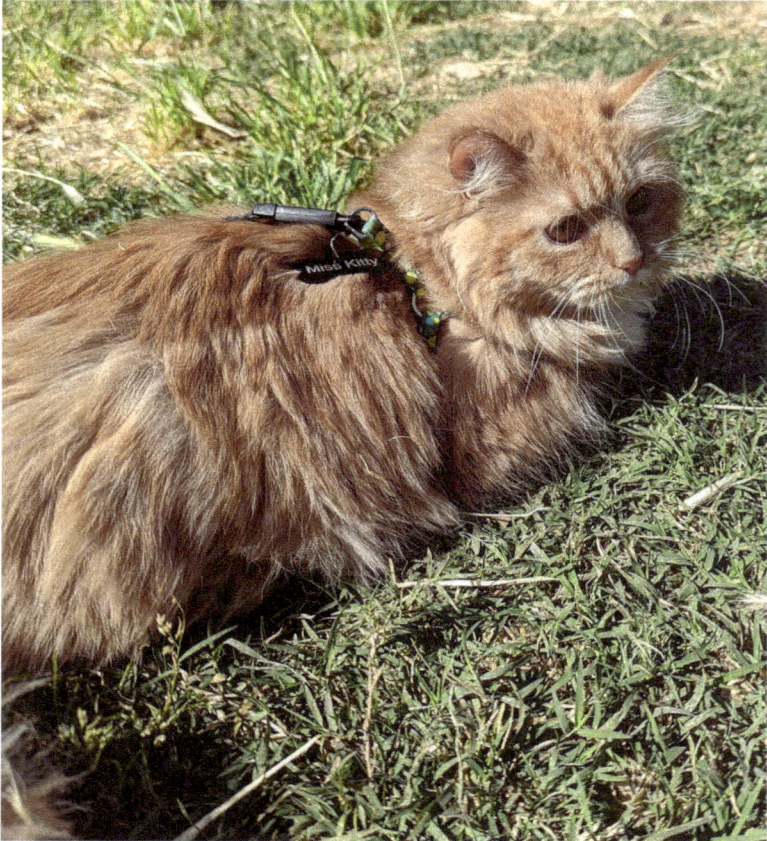

Chapter 11
Ingredients for Health

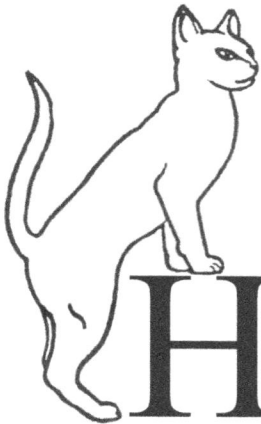

Having information at your fingertips is one of the great things about today's modern age. Included in this chapter are many of the odds and ends that will help you make your own homemade diets for your Miss Kitty. Variety and balance again are key to a healthy and happy kitty. Included are protein sources, taurine levels, definitions and many tricks and tips to help you in your journey to making informed and smart decisions.

Meat Sources Fat Content

From Highest Fat Content to Lowest

Generally based off of a 100g weight. For more information, please see the USDA Food database.

Duck 39	Lamb 23g
Pork 21g	Squab 24g
Goose domestic 34g	Beef 13
Pheasant 9g	Ostrich 9g
Chicken 8g	Venison 7g
Turkey 8g	Rabbit 6g
Veal 7g	Guinea Pig 8g
Emu 4g	Beaver 5g
Quail 5g	Horse 5g
Rabbit (wild) 2g	Kangaroo 1g
Goat 3g	Turkey (wild) 1g

Making Egg Shell Calcium

Eggshell calcium has the great advantage that it is very low in phosphorus. It can be added in amounts that will balance the phosphorus content of the meat. It also avoids the concerns of the potential for lead and mercury some lower quality bovine bone meal products can be contaminated with. You can purchase eggshell calcium or make your own. If you buy it, make sure it is pure eggshells with nothing else added. Many products have added vitamins but are not a complete product and will through your ratios off. Follow the directions on the product for how much to add per pound of meat. The fun part is egg shell calcium is super easy to make. Save the shells from your used eggs but wash the inside out, be sure to leave the membrane intact as best you can, there are lots of additional nutrients you want to save and get use from. Dry them by baking at 300°F for 10 minutes. Grind them in a clean coffee grinder or food processor. Wait for a while, think several minutes, before opening the grinder to let the powder settle. You avoid the cloud of powder coming out that way. One large egg will make around one teaspoon of powder. Store the powder in an air-tight container. Most powder, once finely ground contains between 1900 to 2300 mg of elemental calcium. Since we are aiming for 1000 to 1200 mg per pound of meat in boneless recipes, this means we would add 1/2 teaspoon per pound of meat

What is Muscle Meat, and What is Considered Secreting Organ Meats?

Secreting organs are very rich in many nutrients and should be included in an approximately 10% ratio in homemade diets as previously discussed. If feeding a premix diet, be sure to read the labels carefully.

Muscle	Secreting Organ
Heart	Liver
Gizzard	Kidney
Tongue	Spleen
Lung/Trachea	Sweatbreads*
Green Tripe (not bleached)	Testicles/Brains

*Sweatbreads include thymus and pancreas.

Some Quick Taurine Levels for Reference

Remember, cats are taurine-dependent for proper eye and heart function. You absolutely *must* be sure whatever you feed, in whatever form, has sufficient levels of taurine.

🐾 Cooking/heat processing/long periods of freezing all negatively affect taurine levels.

🐾 Measured as mg of taurine per kg of wet (water included) weight. Below are some of the most common protein sources:

Beef – in general 430 +/-

Ground <30% fat 360 +/-   Liver   190 +/-

Ground<15% fat 398 +/-   Lung   950 +/-

Heart   650 +/-   Spleen 875 +/-

Kidney   225 +/-   Tongue 1250 +/-

Duck   **Rabbit -**

Leg Meat 1780 +/-   Ground Whole 373+/-

Horse in general   325 +/-

Pork Loin   550+/-

Lamb   Kidney 775 +/-

Kidney 240 +/-   Liver 855 +/-

Leg   470 +/-   Lung   775 +/-

Chicken

Breast, Boneless, Skinless	160 +/-
Ground Whole	950+/-
Necks/Backs	575 +/-
Leg	335 +/-
Dark Meat	1600+/-

Turkey

Ground 7% Fat	2005 +/-
Dark Meat	3050+/-
Light Meat	+/-300
Whole Breast w/Portion of Ribs	93 +/-

Remember no measurement is exact due to what the protein source was fed throughout its life prior to it becoming lunch for Miss Kitty.

Also, the smaller the prey source. the higher its heart beat and therefor the more taurine that animal's heart contains.

Some Basic Notes on Ingredients

When using chicken, this protein lacks zinc and thiamine. Be sure your supplement/completer contain this in sufficient quantities

Beef and other ruminant animal organs are critical for copper and iron. Ruminants include cattle, sheep, goats, buffalo, deer, and elk. Other livers such as pork, obviously do contain copper and iron, just in lower quantities.

Chicken livers are good for folate (B-9) which is critical for red cell production.

Beef livers need to be used in moderation as they contain very high levels of Vitamin A which can be toxic over time. Be sure if using this source to mix with other sources or even use a feeding formula that doesn't use it as part of your mix.

One of the biggest reasons to purchase and use completers, should be self-evident. If you want, you can always purchase over 15 individual vitamin and mineral additions, weigh and measure it all out, store it properly, mix it properly, and then hope that Miss Kitty likes it. Completer products are safe, simple and easy to use, because all of that has been done for you. Most such products also have flavorings that are extremely palatable to a wide variety of cats.

Kittens have small stomachs. Kittens should be fed between 4 and 6 small meals a day at minimum, and 8-10 is more optimal when feeding raw. Adults should be fed *no less* than 3 meals a day when feeding raw, and there is evidence that feeding more often and smaller meals is better and more natural. Kittens should be fed in the same range as adults in the 80% meat, 6-10% organ, and between 6 to 10% bone/calcium.

Kittens like children learn early, so offering a wide variety at a young age of protein sources and completer flavors will only benefit both you and your future Miss Kitty.

Kittens should also have a source of DHA in their diets (omega 3's) DHA can be found in cold-water fish like tuna, sardines, salmon, mackerel, whitefish, and herring. Freeze-dried as treats make an easy addition for your kitty, and bonus – the bones are 100% digestible.

Chapter 12
Equipment for Raw Diets

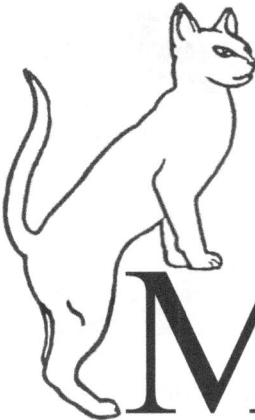

Making homemade cat food isn't hard to do at all. In fact, anyone can, and you can too! Once you start making your own, you'll realize that raw food for cats doesn't have to be complicated. Learning how big companies make theirs, helps to know how ground raw meals are made, because commercially-made frozen foods are created in virtually the same way, just on a much larger scale. You get the peace of mind knowing exactly what is in your best friend's food as well as the satisfaction of having made it yourself. Your household of kitties benefit immensely, your budget benefits from healthier pets, there's less waste to clean up and throw out, and you have a peace of mind that you haven't had before.

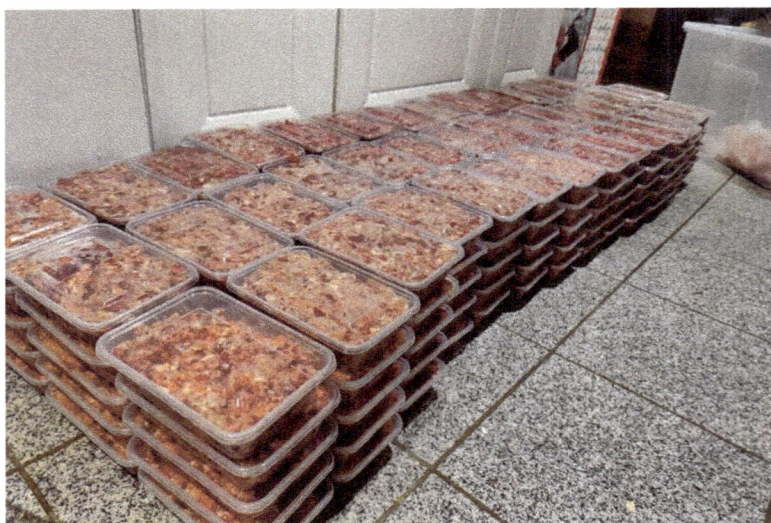

So let's start with some basics. What *exactly* will you need to make your own foods? That partly depends on how involved you want to be with the process. Some folks buy meat grinders, while others use human-grade already-butchered ground meats. Either is an option, but here is a list of what we think most kitchens should have to make their own feline homemade raw diets...

🐾 **A Very Sharp High-Quality Knife**. Seems obvious right? Many of our home kitchens don't have a chef-quality knife. Without one, it will make your job much harder, and you're much more likely to injure yourself on a sub-standard knife edge.

🐾 **Poultry Shears**. For when the knife just isn't enough. Great tool to have handy.

🐾 **Meat Grinder**. Make sure if you do get a grinder, that it is of sufficient quality to handle bones. High-end models can be quite pricey, but will pay for themselves in the long-run if you have a wish to make larger batches. Look for a unit that has a reverse function, since most clogs and jams are caused not by the bones, but by the sinew, skin and cartilage. Having a reverse will save you loads of time. Remember, these units can be quite heavy too, so be careful. Also note that all the parts of a grinder must come apart for good cleaning and sanitizing. Hand-wash only in hot water with a good sanitizer, never use a dishwasher for your grinder parts! Also, some grinders can be noisy, so make sure you are prepared with ear plugs or ear buds in case you need them.

- 🐾 **A Meat Cleaver**. Again, high-quality and very sharp. Not 100% necessary if you aren't working with larger carcasses/pieces, but handy to have in either case.

- 🐾 **A Larger Cutting Board.** No one wants to use their bare counter space for making raw meals. Always put your work on a larger covered area. Even newspaper or butcher paper can be used to cover your work space, then place the cutting board on top of that. Before purchasing, make sure the board will fit in your dishwasher, or you could find yourself in a pickle for cleanup!

- 🐾 **Stainless Steel Mixing Bowls.** Absolutely essential. Can be completely sanitized, can be frozen, heated, and put in the dishwasher. I personally would have a nesting set of three. The smallest to mix your supplements and eggs in separately, the middle one for what comes out of your grinder or what you combine for your primary meats and organs, and the largest to combine the other two into easily to prevent spillage. Stainless steel will last a lifetime, and never wear out or have to be replaced.

- **Kitchen Scale**. Well, obviously! You have to weigh everything right? A lot of folks who make their own do so on a small enough scale (pun intended), that they might not need a super-duper kitchen scale. But it's a good plan to prepare and have one that, at the very least, goes up to 5 lb., and preferably one that can handle up to 10 lb. Even though you may only have one kitty you are preparing meals for, when there is a super sale on that piece of meat, you can save time and money by buying in larger quantities as a general rule.

- **Disposable Gloves.** This might surprise a few folks, but it is always better to be safe than sorry. While our feline friends rarely get food-borne illnesses, we humans are not that lucky. Especially if you are preparing a larger batch of meat and will be spending some time on the preparation portion.

- **Sanitizing Spray.** Now this can be something as simple as bleach, to products that are pet-safe such as Odoban, Lysol, Clorox wipes and many others. Be sure to check your labels.

Your available freezer space will dictate how much homemade raw cat food you can reasonably make and store at a time. So, be sure to do some quick measurements and rearranging prior to starting, or you may find yourself short on space!

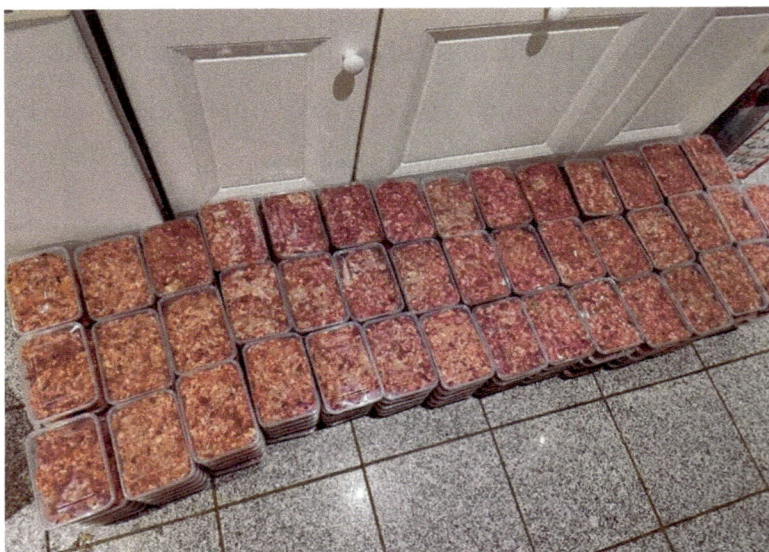

Chapter 13
Basic Recipes

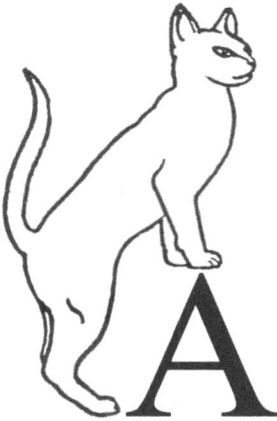

A Few Basic Recipes to Start Your Journey...

So clearly the point of this book is to get you to feed your feline a biologically-appropriate diet of raw meat, bones, organs and supplements. What we aren't going to do is go into a whole lot of preachy recipes. Below you will find a few very basic recipes that hit all the major needs and requirements for your Miss Kitty at home. Part of what we hoped to have gotten across is that variety is not just the spice of life, but the key to making a complete set of diets. Changing protein sources, changing nutrient supplements, and mixing things up, all gives your kitty mental stimulation as well as emotional stimulation. But equally important, it gives you the ability to meet your needs as well. A little short this week on chicken? Fine, add beef. Found some awesome ground turkey on sale? Cool! Neighbor went out hunting and brought back some amazing venison? Jackpot!

These recipes are just starting points. They are not meant to be all-inclusive. As always, rotate your protein sources; rotate your completers; rotate where you get your products from.

We have found that most recipes on the internet are for huge amounts of food. Unless you are feeding a clowder of cats, you simply don't need to make 50 pounds of cat food! It's not practical however cost-effective it may be. It's akin to a single person going to Costco and buying everything by the case and in bulk– "Penny-wise and pound foolish". Plus, most ordinary folks don't have an extra freezer just sitting around to be able to safely store not only the individual items, but the completed product as well.

Often completers offer recipes of their own as well. TCfeline has a basic recipe on their packaging, and a lot of others offer basic recipes on their corresponding websites.

Basic Homemade Raw Diet #1

2 to 3 lb. raw basic boneless proteins

1 lb. raw secondary boneless protein

1-2 cups water (personal preference)

Completer powder- follow instructions on product for amount

5 to 7 ounces raw organs such as liver or kidney

1 raw whole egg

Approx. 12 ounces raw chicken hearts. If you can't source this, add in the equivalent of additional primary protein, also the taurine may then need to be supplemented (added) as well.

Depending on what vitamin mix/completer you choose, you may need to add some form of calcium, preferably in the form of whole bone such as wing tips, necks etc. If not those, then calcium carbonate, which has no phosphorus (this is a good thing and has previously been discussed under egg shell calcium including how to make your own) or a bone meal replacement powder. Add approximately 1000 to 1200 mg of calcium per pound of meat. If using your own egg shell calcium, be sure to have pre-measured.

It is easiest to mix all your dry ingredients separately from your wet ingredients, then combine.

Be sure to separate out into individual meals. You can freeze what you won't use within a couple of days, and thaw as needed.

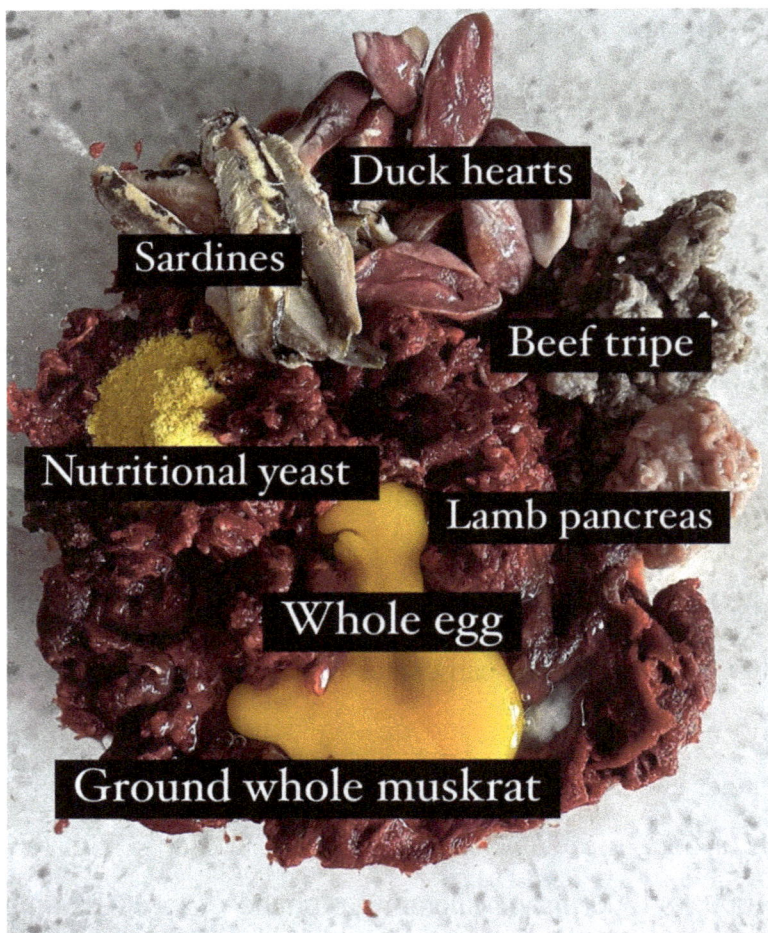

Duck hearts

Sardines

Beef tripe

Nutritional yeast

Lamb pancreas

Whole egg

Ground whole muskrat

Basic Homemade Raw Diet #2

2 to 3 lb. raw basic proteins including bones

1 lb. raw secondary protein including bones

1-2 cups water (personal preference)

Completer powder- follow instructions on product for amount

5 to 7 ounces raw organs such as liver or kidney

1 raw whole egg

Approx. 12 ounces raw chicken hearts. If you can't source this, add in the equivalent of additional primary protein also the taurine may then need to be supplemented (added) as well.

If you are using chicken thighs, legs, or similar items at this point, some of the bones actually should come out of the recipe. Remember, cats need less than 10% overall bones, closer to 6 to 7%. Chicken and turkey lends itself well to being deboned. Ground pork or beef shouldn't contain bones. The remaining bone can easily be ground, especially for younger kittens or older cats. This is where a grinder comes in and is an excellent use.

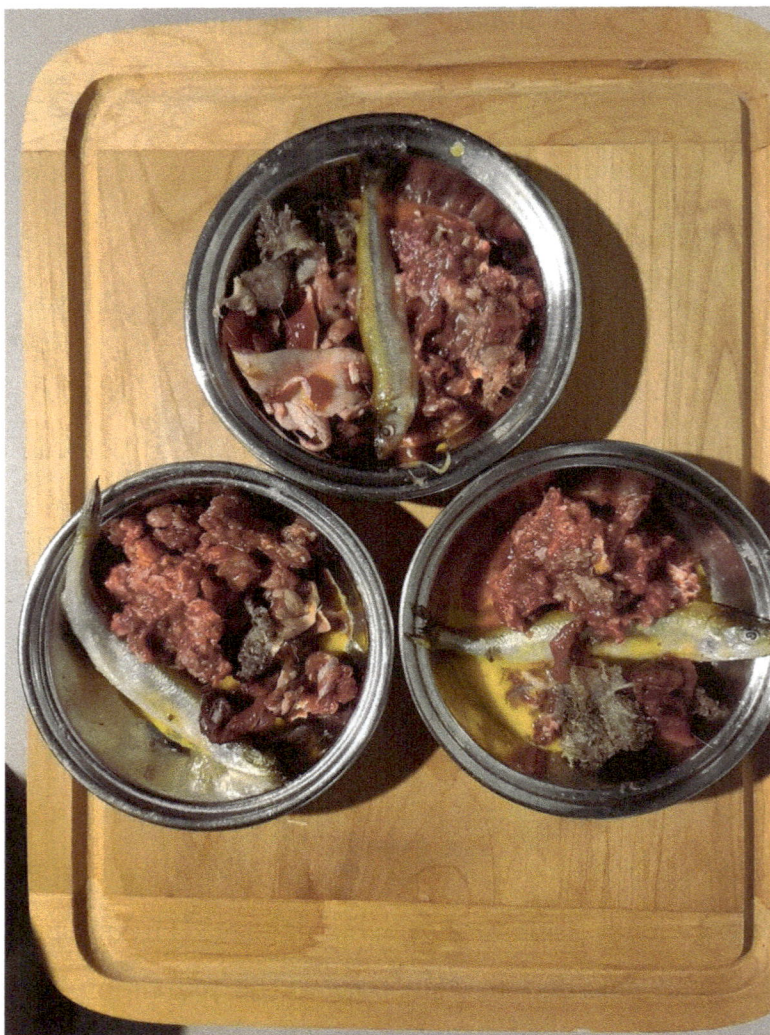

Super Simple Beyond Basic Raw Diet #3

Raw meat either chunked or ground, add in water and a completer that contains calcium and taurine!

If using chunked, be sure Miss Kitty finishes the excess moisture, or the balance will be thrown off.

By using ground, you can ensure all the moisture and mixed completer gets well saturated and distributed, and therefore consumed.

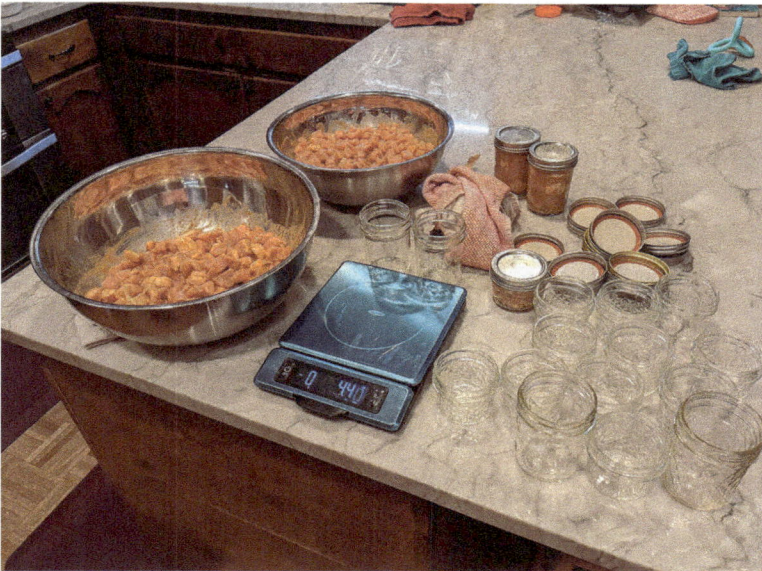

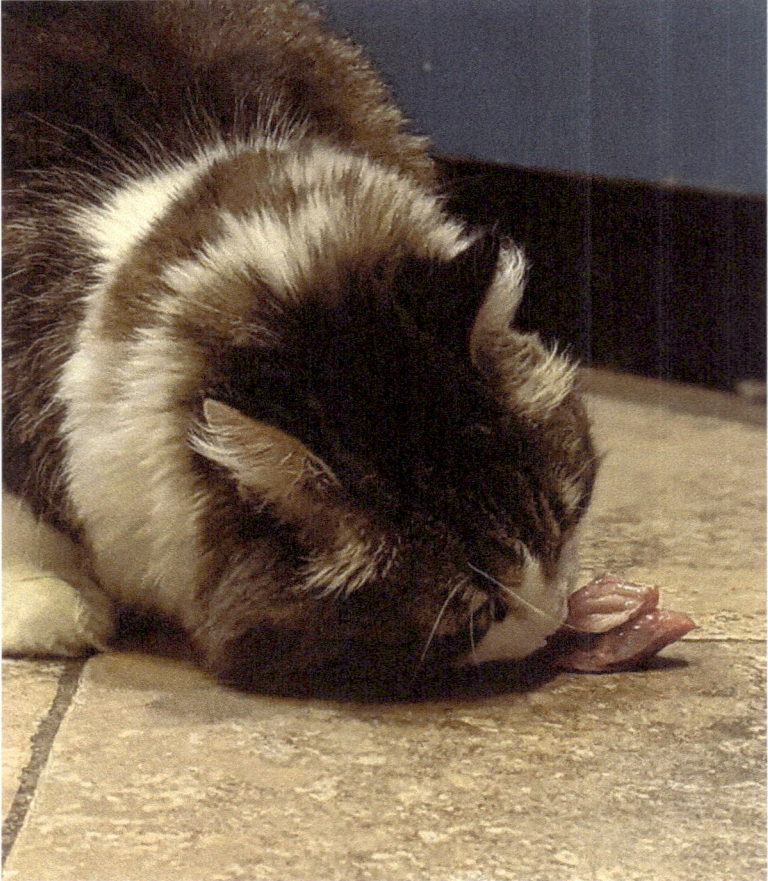

Chapter 14
Be Prepared!

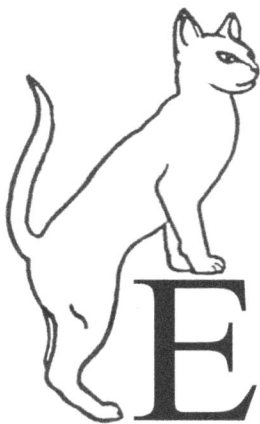

Emergency Preparedness – Don't Be Caught Unawares!

If these last couple of years have taught us anything, it is to *be prepared!* Fires in California caused mass evacuations. Tens of thousands of people had to leave their homes, and some even had to leave their beloved pets. Others left for work that morning, only to be told they couldn't go back into the evacuation zones to retrieve their pets or belongings. Earthquakes in Mexico caused so much damage and destruction that pets simply weren't in the forefront of many people's minds. Hurricanes in the Gulf, tornadoes in the Midwest, and the list goes on.

We have a few recommendations for those scary and hectic times, because let's face it, making the choice of how to feed your cat might have to take a bit of a sideways slide during a mass evacuation when your very life could be on the line. But that doesn't mean it has to be a world of unknown for Miss Kitty.

During your "normal" life; those times when you are bored and nothing extraordinary is happening, there are still things you can passively do to help pave the way to safety and security for your beloved feline.

Always have a crate out with its door open and a soft bed inside. Just like training a puppy that the crate is a safe space, this also helps Miss Kitty be less afraid, and even comfortable in the crate. It doesn't become a foreign and frightening object. Remember that cats run to those "safe places" in times of distress just like dogs. Make this one of those "safe places". Play in and around the crate with a hand-held wand toy. Feed treats in the crate itself. And move the crate from time to time, first under the table, then by the stairs, then around the front door. This is called conditioning, and is something so simple and so crucial, should you need it.

I should mention that we are talking about a hard-sided plastic crate, with a metal door. Soft-sided crates provide literally zero protection in exigent circumstances. Your precious pet needs all the protection it can get. You may be running, bouncing the crate, crushing a soft purse-style carrier, objects can fall in a vehicle on top of the soft-style carrier, again crushing Miss Kitty. And flying objects from a hurricane or tornado become nothing but projectiles and missiles to a pet in a soft-sided carrier. Hard plastic with a metal door is truly the only way to help ensure your pet is protected.

We are talking about having raw food available to feed your kitty. Maybe lines of travel are shut down due to tornado damage. Or perhaps due to civil unrest, folks like Amazon and UPS refuse to service an area for a few days or more.

What about having to stay in a hotel that might not have a refrigerator? All of these are circumstances that can occur and in fact, *have* occurred just in the last couple of years.

Hopefully, throughout the course of this book, it has been made abundantly clear that variety is the spice of life. Well, variety may also be the key to not having to sacrifice your cat's health during times of distress. All of these situations are scary and disturbing enough. The last thing you need is a sick kitty who went from a perfect world of homemade raw diets to subsisting on kibble. Well, I am here to tell you it doesn't have to happen. It shouldn't happen. And it is entirely within your ability to make sure things are done right. Reading through this book, you've learned *why* you feed raw foods. You've learned *how* to make your own foods. And you've learned Miss Kitty needs to be fed multiple times a day. But how does any of this help in an emergency? Simple – always without fail, make one of those meals freeze-dried raw. Pick a brand your kitty likes through trial and error. Once you've found the brand that pleases Miss Kitty, buy an extra bag (or two), if you have more than Miss Kitty in your care. Leave them sealed and place them securely in an additional airtight Ziploc bag. Place this bag in your emergency crate. And always have these items on hand, ready to go at a moment's notice. It is fast, simple, clean, and sanitary. It is bug-proof and water proof!

The other thing to consider is a bottle of water. Clean, safe water is also imperative in such emergency situations. Now, when that sudden emergency rears its ugly head, Miss Kitty can rely on you to still be able to provide her some measure of comfort and consistency. This will help her health to stay stable during trying times, as well as her psychological comfort, all from you preparing the shelf-stable safe food she is familiar with.

140

Chapter 15

Diet Retailers

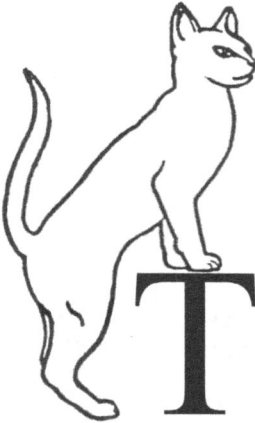

This is not a complete list by any means, and neither the author nor the publisher is endorsing any one brand or type over another. endorsing any one brand or type over another.

Each cat is unique and individual and what works for one cat even within the same household, may not work for another. Trial and error are your friend here. This is just about options.

Currently Reliable Sources of Raw Meat Diets and Preparations for Felines

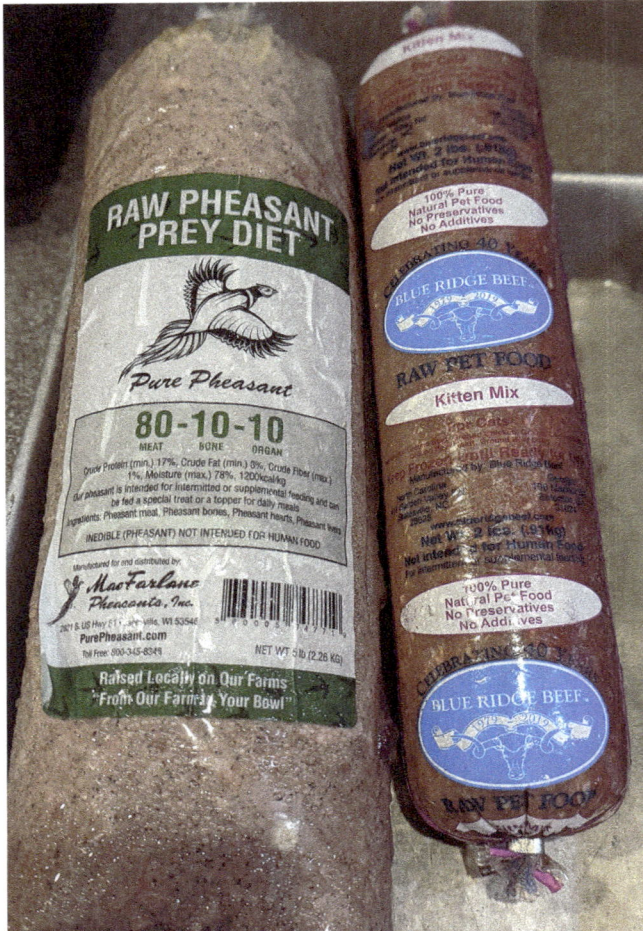

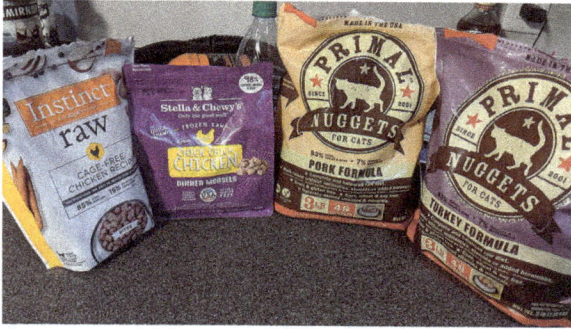

Frozen Raw Meals Only

Answers Pet Food (One of the only companies out there to legally challenge the FDA mandates and the AAFCO cooperation of unlawful standards for raw foods.)
https://www.answerspetfood.com/

Blue Ridge Beef
https://blueridgebeef.com/

Bobcat Raw
(Offers a subscription service of fresh raw diets.)
https://bobcatrawfood.com/

Meat Me
(Human-Grade Meats out of Canada)
https://www.meatme.ca

Pure Pheasant by MacFarlane Pheasants
https://www.purepheasant.com

Savage Cat Food
https://savagecatfood.com/

Tiki Cat
(Now makes a frozen raw variety of diets.)
https://tikipets.com/cat/

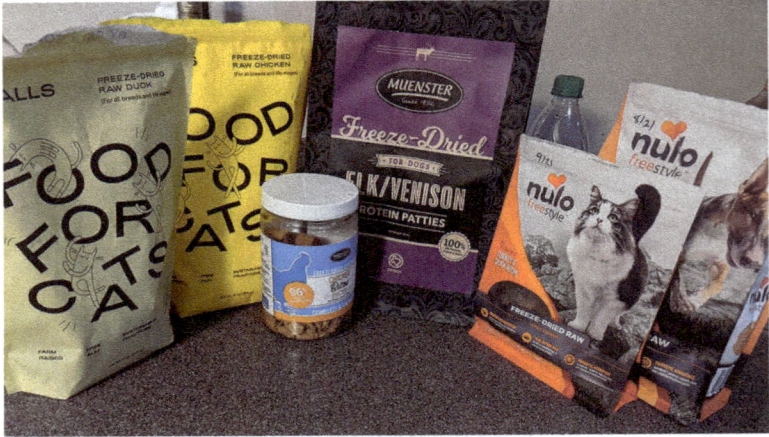

Both Frozen and Freeze-Dried Raw Meals

Instinct
https://instinctpetfood.com/cat/

Northwest Naturals
https://nw-naturals.net/

Stella & Chewy's
https://www.stellaandchewys.com

Vital Cat
https://www.vitalessentialsraw.com/cat/food/

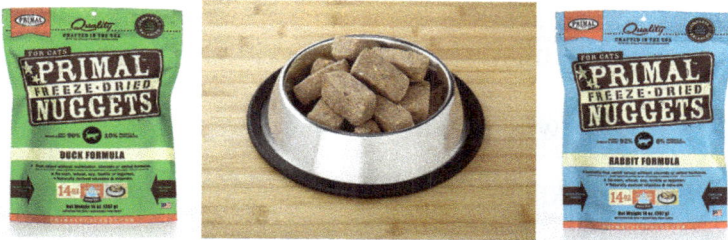

Freeze-Dried Raw Meals Only

Feline Natural
(From New Zealand)
https://www.k9natural.com/cat-food-range/

Meat Mates
(Also from New Zealand)
https://meatmates.com/meow-dinner/

Nulo
(Offers freeze dried raw meals but not frozen ones)
https://nulo.com/

Primal Pet Foods
(These folks also carry fresh goat's milk.)
https://primalpetfoods.com/

Purpose Pet Foods
(Offers freeze-dried raw meals but not frozen)
https://purposepetfood.com/

This is just a "short list". Go onto Facebook and I am sure you will be inundated with dozens of branded foods, including raw and freeze-dried.

Amazon will have more without fail. One of the things about this list is that none of them are a subscription service. You can buy any of these individual products from any number of retailers across the internet.

I despise subscription services. That in no way implies that their products are not good, I am sure many are. But a subscription service often means being locked into a certain protein source at a much higher cost. And remember, one of the keys is variety.

Another thing to not overlook is some items that are also labeled for usage in dogs. Sadly, dogs are a larger share of the market, so from a company's point of view it makes sense to market to the larger potential.

However, there are several companies who make single-ingredient products that are freeze dried, frozen, or fresh. Some pictures (including those on pages 142-145) have been included in this book to give you an idea of what you can look for. Always look carefully before using a product labeled for another species.

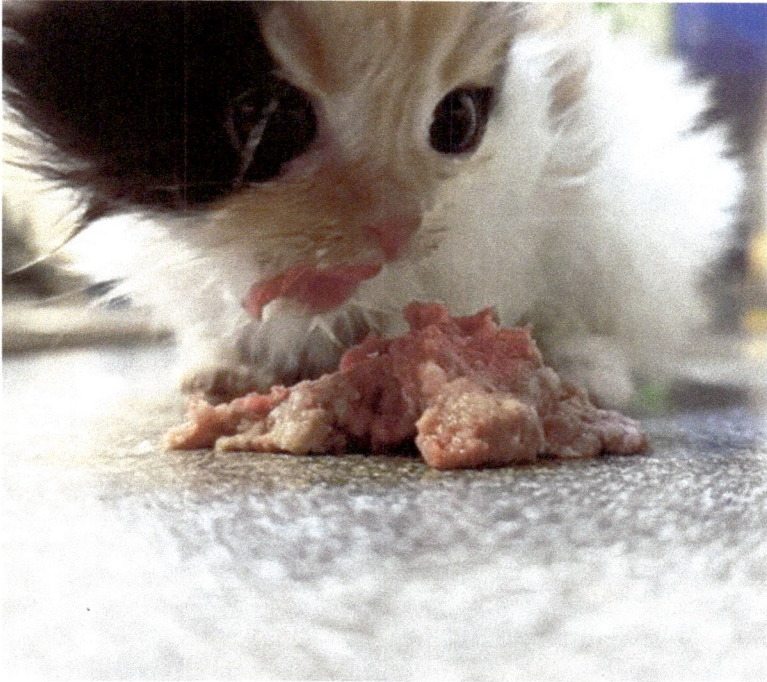

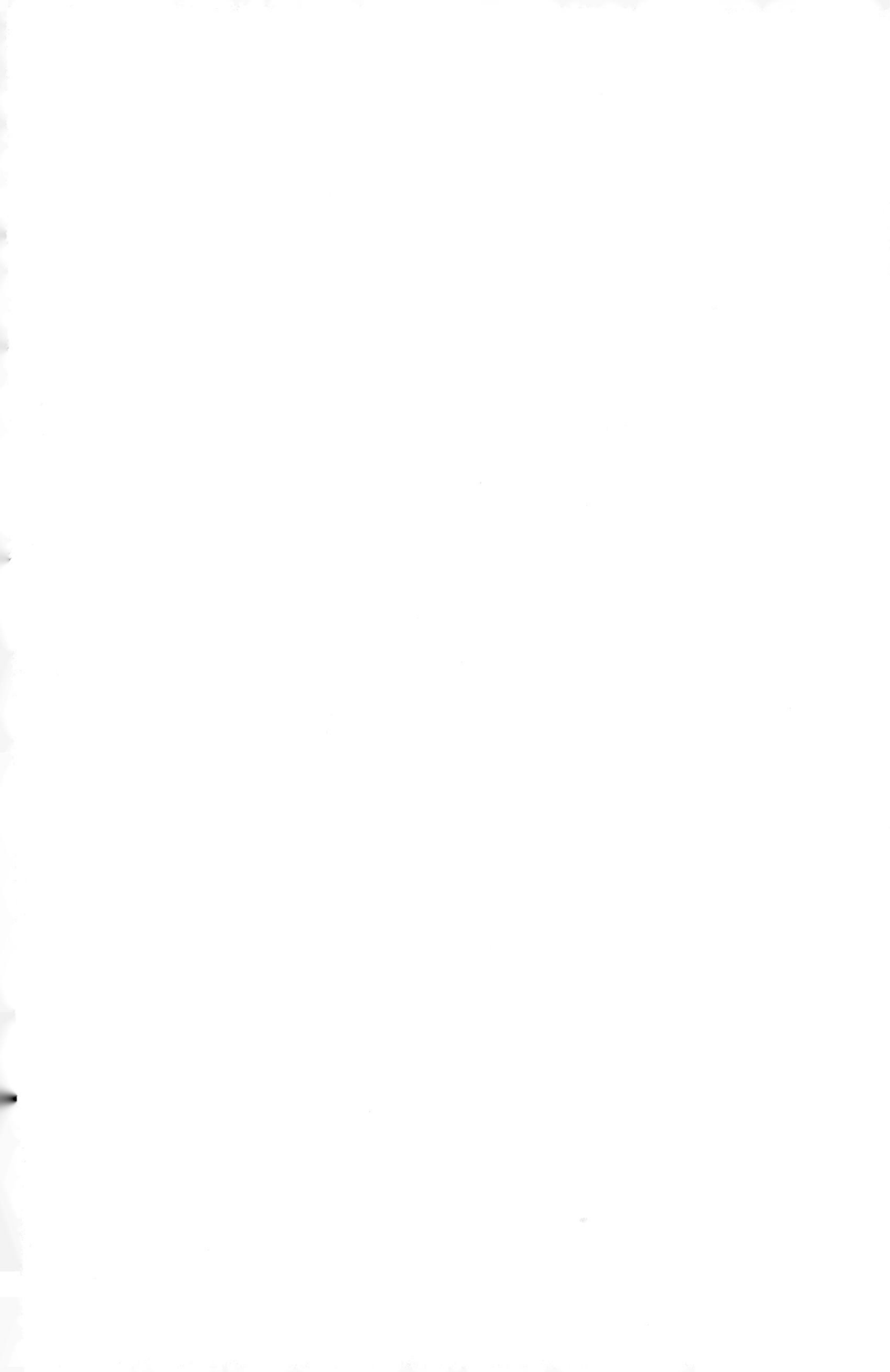

www.ingramcontent.com/pod-product-compliance
Lightning Source LLC
Chambersburg PA
CBHW070935030426
42336CB00014BA/2688